I Miss You, Daddy!

I Miss You, Daddy!

Anthony D. Luck

Writers Club Press
San Jose New York Lincoln Shanghai

I Miss You, Daddy!

Writers Club Press
an imprint of iUniverse, Inc.

For information address:
iUniverse, Inc.
5220 S. 16th St., Suite 200
Lincoln, NE 68512
www.iuniverse.com

The information in this book is written from the personal perspective of the author, and is intended for informational use only.

ISBN: 0-595-22973-5

Printed in the United States of America

To my beloved father Marcellus Heywood Luck, Jr.,
October 1, 1924 to July 28, 1988.

To my brother Marcellus Heywood Luck III,
July 28, 1947 to May 2, 1994.

And to my sister Mary Ann Luck,
February 5, 1949 to December 3, 1996.

They have all fallen asleep in death, two of them due to cancer.

To my wife Shirley Anne, with whom I plan on spending the rest of my life,
and my children Stacey Leigh, Peter Alexander, Stephen Anthony, and
Nicholas Ian. I will always cherish, remember, and love them.
I am determined to spend as much time now with them as I possibly can.

And finally,

To the rest of my family—Jackie, Rick, Andy, Marcy, Roxy, Sue, and our
beloved mother. I love you all very much.

Contents

Introduction

◆

The Death Of A Loved One

My father died on July 28, 1988 opening a gaping wound in my heart that today, years later, is only now very slowly beginning to heal. Since my dear father's death over 13 years ago, I have gone through all of the emotional reactions of someone who has just lost a loved one. The death of someone you love, especially a parent, is like losing a part of yourself. I felt:

- SHOCK—How in the world could something like this possibly have happened? How could my father be dead? What is life going to be like without a father, MY father?

- DISBELIEF—No! He's not really gone! He just can't be dead! He has always been there for us! He has always been the strong one!

- EMOTIONAL NUMBNESS—A strange feeling that I simply stopped functioning, that life as I knew it simply ceased to exist. I could no longer feel anything emotionally, and I couldn't think about anything else.

- ANGER—I was angry with the doctors and the nurses who let my father die. I was angry with friends or relatives who said or did the wrong things while trying to comfort me. I was angry with myself for not being there for my father when he needed me. I was angry with myself for all the times I had failed to listen to my father, and I was angry with myself for not telling my father how much I love him.

- GUILT—I couldn't help recalling all the times I had been angry, or less than patient with my father. I couldn't help recalling the times I had not treated my beloved father with the respect that he deserved. I couldn't even tell him before he died how much I love him! What was wrong with me?

Most of all, I continually fought feelings of deep loneliness, and a sadness that seemingly would never end. I was unable to even look at a picture of my father.

As the years passed, I was unable to think about the loss of my father, or even to discuss it, until now—

Acknowledgements

This part of the book is very difficult for me. I owe so many people so much, for taking care of us, for being there when we needed them, and for inspiring the contents of this book. I am afraid that I might overlook someone, but I want to at least try to thank as many people as possible, and to express my heartfelt gratitude.

My family has always been an unlimited source of strength, comfort and financial support. My wife Shirley has always been there for me, with me, every step of the way. My children, although I feel that they are having a hard time dealing with the potential loss of their father, are doing very well with encouragement and support. My mom who brought me into the world, my brothers, sisters, nieces, etc. are always there for me. Whatever I need, and whenever I need it, to the extent of their ability, they provide it. Their moral support has also been very encouraging. This would include a hand-made, from the heart, Get-Well card that I received from a niece while in the hospital. This card was very appreciated, and arrived just when I needed a boost in spirits.

Thanks to the doctors, the nurse practitioner, the nursing staff, and the Social Worker at Shadyside Hospital in Pittsburgh, PA. where I spent a lot of my time. They explained every procedure, every drug, everything I had to undergo. They helped to assuage every fear that we had. They were very caring and considerate, and helped my wife and I through the tough times we were soon to experience.

Many thanks to the doctors, the nurses and staff of Pennsylvania Hospital in Philadelphia, PA, where my wife and I had to go for a peripheral stem cell transplant without the use of blood. They were there through the whole procedure, ever watchful, ever considerate. When my red count had dropped to about 5, they patiently explained to my wife and I what I was going through, and what to expect. They watched me closely when I had heart and breathing problems, and treated my wife and I like honored guests, or visiting royalty, rather than patients.

Thanks also to the Center for Bloodless Medicine and Surgery at Pennsylvania Hospital in Philadelphia, who assisted in making the many arrangements for us in Philadelphia. This included travel, hotel, food, and other accommodations. They were also there every day while my wife and I were in the hospital, providing encouragement and support, making sure that all of our questions and concerns were being addressed.

I also wish to express my thanks to the following organizations:

- The Corporate Angel Network, who provided free air transportation for my wife and I to Philadelphia, and free air transportation back if, and when, we needed it.

- The Leukemia Society of America, who provided financial assistance for medication, travel for treatment, etc. They also provided very informative brochures on cancer, and always asked if there was anything else they could do for us.

- The American Cancer Society and the International Myeloma Foundation, both of whom continually provide valuable information about treatments, medication, etc. for Multiple Myeloma, via weekly e-mails.

- The Hospital Liaison Committee and the Hospital Information Systems, both of whom were instrumental in working with my doctors in providing necessary treatments without the use of blood, and in helping us to get through the difficult times.

I would like to thank my spiritual brothers and sisters in the congregations of Jehovah's Witnesses in Pittsburgh and Philadelphia, who were there almost daily in the hospitals in Pittsburgh and in Philadelphia, providing financial, moral, and emotional support. This would include one young teenage sister who, after school and on her own, came to the hospital to spend time with me, to talk to me and read to me the latest issue of the Watchtower magazine.

I sincerely hope that I have not overlooked anyone. If I have, it was certainly not intentional. There have just been so many people involved in our lives, helping us, providing financial, emotional, and spiritual support. If I have overlooked anyone, I am sincerely sorry. I am so grateful to everyone who has assisted us, and is continuing to assist us. Thank you, all of you, for all that you have done, and continue to do, in our behalf.

Preface

Anthony D. Luck, happily married husband and father of four children, comes from a close family of three brothers and four sisters. When he heard the news that his beloved father was stricken with cancer and was about to die, it seemed as if his whole world had just been turned upside down. The potential loss of a parent is truly devastating. His father died not long after that, in 1988.

Then, in 1999, Anthony got the devastating news that he had Multiple Myeloma, an incurable form of bone cancer. He was also informed that Multiple Myeloma was the same cancer that took the life of his father, just eleven years ago. At the time, he was employed as an Assistant Director for the Housing Authority City of Pittsburgh. How does he tell his employer? More importantly, how does he tell his wife, his children, and his family?

This book is the story of life with, and then without, his beloved father. It is also about Anthony's struggle with Multiple Myeloma, and the assistance provided by doctors, nurses, hospital staff, family, friends, and a host of others. It is a story of courage, of never giving up, no matter what. It is a story of reliance on the strongest power in the universe, that of our Loving Heavenly Father. The book concludes with ten things that cancer patients, their family and friends should know, told from first hand knowledge gained during Anthony's struggle with Multiple Myeloma. This book is also a testament to the strength of love—love of family, love of friends, love of God, and love of life! By sharing what he has learned from his ongoing struggle with Multiple Myeloma, and his fight to survive, Anthony hopes that this book will encourage other cancer survivors and their families, including those like him who have been told there is no cure, and that there is only so much more time to live.

1

The Day That My Father Died

It was 5:45pm, and I was finally staggering through the door of my home, at the end of yet another uneventful day. I had just completed a long, hard day at work, towards the end of an extremely rough week. Now at home, I was at last able to take off my tie and dress clothes, and YES, those extremely uncomfortable dress shoes, and get comfortable! I slipped on my favorite t-shirt and shorts, and a comfortable pair of sandals. I was heading toward my favorite reclining chair in the living room to watch television, with a large bowl of freshly popped, buttered and ever so lightly salted popcorn. That warm buttery popcorn smell just drifted ever so gently up to my nose, causing my mouth to water. I also had a tall, refreshing, ice-cold glass of tea that was beckoning to me from the coffee table. I was just about to lose myself once again in the television world of science fiction, when the telephone rang. "Hello?" I said half-heartedly, hoping that it was a wrong number. "Tony? It's daddy," my sister cried. "He is dying!! The doctors say that over 80% of his bones are cancerous. His bones are so thin now that, if his heart stops, they will be unable to perform CPR. The paddles would go right through his rib cage. We are all going to go out to see him. In fact, I am driving out today. Do you want to go with me?" "Sure, I can leave immediately! Pick me up on your way out!" I replied. I hung up the phone and just stood there, motionless. "This can't be!" I thought. "My father, dying? It just can't be!!" Television, popcorn, iced tea, were all forgotten. I was losing my father!

Slowly, I walked up the steps to tell my wife and children what was happening to my father, and why I needed to be there with him. Then, my wife helped me to pack a suitcase for the long, very difficult trip to see my father, my dear father, for the last time! My sister soon arrived outside, and started blowing the horn for me. So, after saying goodbye to my wife and children, I placed my suitcase in the back of her car, hopped in the front seat, and we began the long, difficult trip to Atlanta, Georgia to say our last goodbyes to our father, the one man who we all thought would never die!! My sister and I drove for hours without saying a word to each other. All we could think of was our father. We just couldn't believe it! Our father was dying!

During the trip, I reflected back to better times with my father, times when he had helped me, times when he was there for me, and the times when I needed him. After a long, 17-hour drive on unfamiliar highway, we arrived safely in Atlanta. We searched for the hospital that was taking care of our father, and then quickly, quietly, we looked for a place to park the car. Then, fearfully, we entered the elevator and pushed the button for my father's floor. As the elevator door opened, we slowly walked toward my father's room, not knowing what to expect, hoping that this was all just a very bad dream. It had to be a dream. Our father would get better, and return home to us.

As we gradually opened the door to the hospital room, we saw our other brothers, sisters, and my niece, gathered around my father's bed. Jackie, Brother, Mary Ann, Ricky, Tony, Andy, Marcy, Roxy, and Sue. We were all there, all of the children, staring in total disbelief. Our father, our "Rock of Gibraltar", was just lying there in a hospital bed, in a coma, with tubes in his nose and in his mouth. Yes, THIS was the strong parent, the one that had always been there for us, the one parent who we thought would NEVER die—and he was dying! I just stood there, speechless. I wanted so desperately to say, "Daddy, I love you! We are all here for you, so just hang in there! Please, Daddy, don't leave us! Don't die!" The words choked up in my throat, and just wouldn't come out. All I could think of were the years of love, tenderness, and unselfish giving that my father had provided. He had always been there for us, providing help and assistance whenever we needed it.

Now, HE needed help, and there was absolutely NOTHING I could do! I watched my father lying there in a coma, and, about an hour after I arrived at the hospital, my father died. I just sat there in the hospital room, refusing to accept it. This just didn't happen! It couldn't happen! It's just not possible! I was standing in a hospital room, surrounded by my brothers and sisters, yet I felt empty, helpless, and very alone!

My mom and dad had separated years prior to this. My dad had remarried and moved to Atlanta, GA. My mom was now living in California. Someone had to call her and tell her that Daddy was dead. I picked up the phone and slowly, painfully, dialed the number. The phone rang several times, and then it was picked up. "Hello?" I could hear my mother's voice on the other end of the line. How could I tell her? "Mom," I said, "this is Tony. I am at the hospital with Dad. Daddy's—" My whole body suddenly went numb, and my mouth stopped working. That word just wouldn't come out! I couldn't even force myself to speak it! My mouth was open, but the words choked up in my throat. I could not tell Mom that Daddy was dead, because he wasn't! He just couldn't be! He's **not** dead! My hands slowly dropped to my lap, and I just sat there, staring at the hospital wall. Ricky, my older brother, slowly took the phone from my hand, and he attempted to tell mom about dad. He also told her that we were all very sorry that she could not be there with us, so that we could comfort her, and hold her. The entire family needed to be together at a time like this. I could hear her screaming and crying on the other end. As my brother Ricky slowly hung up the phone, we made our way from the hospital room, slowly, methodically, stabbed at the heart at the loss of our father. One word repeated itself in my mind over and over again—**WHY**? A hospital priest, hoping to comfort the family, said to us, "Don't worry. Your father has gone to a better place. God has called him to heaven." I couldn't help wondering to myself, why would a loving God **take** a father away from his wife and children?

We stayed in Atlanta long enough to make the necessary arrangements to bury our father. In the days that followed, as we made the necessary funeral arrangements, I didn't cry. All I could think of was that my father was gone. I was dazed, confused, but, for some reason, I couldn't cry. First, we made arrangements for funeral services, and discussed the wording for the funeral announcements. Then, we made the very difficult trip to the cemetery to make the necessary burial arrangements. The hardest thing that we had to do was to select a casket, destined to be the final resting place for our father. Funeral arrangements, cemetery plot, casket, all for my father? I still could not believe it! As we walked through looking at the caskets, reality finally hit home. Our father was dead, really dead, and there was nothing we could do. When the arrangements had been completed, my father's body was delivered to the funeral home that we had selected for preparation. Then, the family was asked to come to the funeral home to review the preparations made prior to the funeral.

At the funeral home, when my older brother Ricky saw our beloved father in the casket for the first time, it was just too much for him to bear. He grabbed hold of the casket and wouldn't let go. He didn't say anything—not one sound came out of his mouth—yet, tears were streaming down his face. I could only imagine how he must have felt. Ricky and my dad had been more like brothers than father and son. He had spent the last few months before my father died, using his laptop computer to research the disease that was killing my father. He had looked up every possible medication, herb, or supplement that could keep him alive, every possible treatment, and every potential ray of hope. Though some of the research had looked promising, nothing, absolutely nothing, had worked. My father had finally agreed to go to the hospital much too late, and the disease had progressed too far to be stopped. Plus, the procedures and medications known for treatment of Multiple Myeloma were not as advanced as they are today. So, now our father was dead. I wanted to cry, but I couldn't. I just stood there looking at my father—dead, unreachable, alone.

During the funeral services, my sisters all cried uncontrollably. They just couldn't stop. The loss of their father, the funeral services, all of this caused a deep emotional void that could not be filled. A deep, painful sorrow was welling up inside of me, caused by the loss of my father, and the pain felt by my brothers and sisters. Again, I wanted to cry, but I just couldn't. I just sat there dazed, not seeing, not speaking, and not hearing. Then, as daddy's casket was slowly lowered into the ground, we all realized that this was it! The last glimpse of our beloved father, our last goodbye. Our father, our beloved father, was gone! My sisters cried and screamed, "Daddy, daddy, no, no!" I agonized inside, but still, I could not cry. My father was now in a box that was being lowered into a hole that was being filled with dirt. He was dead and gone, and I still could not believe it! After the funeral, we were driven to the Hall reserved for family and friends to get together after the funeral services, in several of the long black limousines that they provided. Sitting in the back seat of one of the limousines, I happened to glance down at the picture of my father on one of the notices provided during the funeral services. This was the man we had just seen buried under a pile of dirt, the father who had once been very vibrant, and very much alive. This was MY father, the father that I so desperately wanted to come back!

Then, for the first time, a flood of tears came that I couldn't stop, that I didn't WANT to stop! My father was gone, GONE, and I could not bring him back. I cried for my father. I cried for my mother, my brothers and sisters, and, finally, I cried for me! The days of anger, frustration, remorse and sadness that I had pent up inside could no longer be contained. I wept for what seemed like an eternity, but the pain, the emptiness, would not go away. I just could not stop crying. The thought of life without my father in it was just too much to bear. We stopped to get something to eat, but I could not eat. I couldn't stop crying. There was no sound, just an unrelenting stream of tears from my eyes. My sister Mary Ann came over to me and said that I needed to try and eat something, so I tried to eat through the tears. For me, the remainder of the day was full of sadness, loneliness, and remorse. I couldn't think of anything but my father. That evening, my sister Marcy wore my father's favorite jacket, and fell asleep in his favorite chair, hoping that he might return from the dead, so that she could see him, and perhaps even speak to him, one last time. Yet, he didn't come back, he couldn't come back, for he was gone!

Several months after the funeral, I drove with my wife and children back to Atlanta, GA to meet with my brothers and sisters, and my uncles Randy and Oliver. It was great for us to be able to get together again, this time under a little more favorable circumstances. We were able to talk more about what was happening in our lives. I had not seen my uncles in a while, so we had a lot of catching up to do. It was very difficult for me to look at Uncle Randy, because he looked and sounded so much like my father. I loved my uncle, and I knew that he was hurting too, for he had just lost his brother. We all enjoyed dinner together, talked for a while, and then went to bed. It had been a long day. The next morning, after breakfast, our stepmother called all of us into our father's bedroom. She explained, "I called all of you in here because Marcellus and I wanted his clothes to go to the family". She had all of his shirts and pants laid out on the bed, and his shoes were at the foot of the bed. His coats, jackets, and hats were hanging in an open closet. She then continued, "Before he died, your father said to make sure that Tony has the first pick of his clothes. He knew that Tony is quiet and won't speak up for himself. If I don't let him go first, he'll wait until everyone else has selected". The tears came all over again, because my dad KNEW me so well! He loved each and every one of his children. Now, he was no longer here with us, to hug, to thank, or to love. Yet, even while dying, he was thinking about his children. He was thinking about me! I didn't think that I would ever get over that empty feeling of losing someone you deeply loved. Even for a year or two after his death, every time I saw a funeral, saw someone die on television, or even when the word "death" was mentioned, I cried over the loss of my father. Even while watching the movie, *King*

Kong Lives! when King Kong lay dying, holding his son in his hand, I started crying all over again.

Now, over thirteen years later, I still cry from time to time when I think about my father. The pain, the hurt, is still there. My father is gone, but I can remember the good times we had as a family. In fact, I can just imagine how my father must have felt when it was MY turn to come into the world—

2

Childhood Years With My Father

My life began in the womb of my mommy sometime in December 1952. Mommy was excited when she heard the news from her doctor, but she was afraid of how daddy might react, for this was their fifth child. Mommy did not work, and daddy already had three jobs, counting the army reserves. So, when daddy found out, he was very upset! "We are barely making ends meet now! What are we going to do?" he exclaimed. Mommy didn't have an answer. She just sat there, quietly, while daddy fumed. "We can't afford another baby! It's just not possible!" Yet, inside mommy's womb, I was beginning to grow.

8 WEEKS OLD

After about 7 ½ weeks of pregnancy, mommy could see and feel visible evidence of my existence. I actually began to move around inside her womb. At eight weeks of age, all of my body parts were in place—arms, legs, tiny fingers and toes. I had increased in length about 240 times, and my weight had grown to a million times more than at conception. I am grateful that this growth rate will not continue after I am born, for I would become huge! The watery sac that my mommy provided for me gives me a cushioned, temperature-controlled play-room in which to tumble and play. This playing around will strengthen muscles that I will need once I am outside the weightless-ness of this bag of water. I can't wait until my mommy and daddy can actually see me!

16 WEEKS OLD

Wow! I am now 16 weeks old! About 3 weeks ago my taste buds started functioning, so now I can tell when mommy eats something sweet. I *really* kick up a fuss when she eats something yucky, like lima beans. YUK!! Mommy doesn't know it yet, but I have started to suck my thumb. To a limited extent, I can see, hear, taste, smell and feel in my little world.

7 MONTHS OLD

Mommy has been talking to me every day now, and, every night before she goes to bed, she sings me a lullaby. I think she has a beautiful voice! I try to sing along with her, but only bubbles come out. Daddy has been watching mommy's belly getting bigger and bigger as I grow gradually inside of her. He tenderly rubs her belly, waiting to feel the movement of his child. He doesn't know yet that I am a boy, but I heard him tell mom that he didn't care whether their new baby was a little boy or a little girl, as long as the baby inside is healthy and strong. He didn't want another child at first, but now, he couldn't wait for the arrival of his new baby. I can't wait to snuggle deep within his chest as he holds me, safe and warm, in his strong arms!

9 MONTHS OLD

Finally, I am on my way! Mommy's contractions are coming closer together, and daddy is shaking as he attempts to call the hospital. Boy, is he nervous! Daddy quickly grabs mommy's packed suitcase and helps her into the station wagon. Then, off we race to the hospital. What fun! Daddy is going through stop signs and red lights. We must be going a zillion miles an hour! When we finally get to the hospital, mommy and I are whisked away in a wheelchair, as daddy is kept busy filling out hospital forms. We arrived at the hospital at around 11:45pm. Then, at 8:43am on October 11, 1953 I decided to come into the world, all 7lb., and 3 oz. Mommy, sweating, tired, but very happy, looks at me for the very first time. "You are so tiny, with little wrinkled hands and feet, but you are so beautiful, Anthony Dean Luck!" Wow! I heard my name mentioned for the first time, and I like it! Daddy seems to like the name too. He looks at me, gives me a big smile, and says, "My son, Anthony Dean Luck!" My parents seem to be so nice! Can I pick them or what? I feel very safe now, protected by two loving parents. I settled down comfortably into my mommy's arms and fall peacefully asleep.

A few hours later, I slowly open my eyes, and mommy and daddy are still there! Then, I notice that I have this strange looking cap on my head, and some soft funny things on my hands and feet. Daddy is the first person to speak to me. "Well, how are you little buddy?" What, "Little Buddy?" Who is "Little Buddy?" They must have changed my name while I was asleep! I really liked being called Anthony. Whose big idea was it to change my name to "Little Buddy"? Then, I hear mommy speaking, "It looks like little Anthony is hungry. Do you want something to eat, Anthony?" Whew, my name is still Anthony! I guess "Little Buddy" is a daddy name. Mommy knows what my real name is, and more importantly, she also has the right idea! I am very hungry! Mommy picks me up, gently supporting my head (that thing is too big for ME to hold up) puts this big, soft, pink thing in my mouth, and something very delicious comes out! I get my first taste of mother's milk, and it is very good. It is much better than that stuff I tasted in the womb. Mommy is so soft and warm; it's hard to stay awake as I finish my first meal in the outside world. Hunger satisfied, I drift peacefully to sleep once again.

This continues for, it seems like forever, but, finally, mommy and I are released from the hospital. Daddy is waiting outside for us in the station wagon. The ride home *from* the hospital is a lot different than the ride *to* the hospital. Daddy is driving a lot slower now. I guess he doesn't want to damage his precious cargo—his lovely wife, and his brand new son! When we finally arrive home, poor daddy doesn't even get a chance to hold his own son, because everyone else wants to—grandparents, neighbors, and four other kids that they tell me are part of my family. But, just before mommy puts me into bed for the night, daddy walks into the room, picks me up in his strong arms, and holds me very close. Looking deep into my eyes, he says, "I love you, Anthony. I am very glad you are here!" I realize, right then and there, that I love him more than anything! I hope to be with him forever! Extremely happy, I once again drift peacefully off to sleep.

1 YEAR OLD

I am now one year old, and I have two sisters and two brothers—Jackie, Brother, Mary Ann and Ricky. I could understand clearly what they were saying but, for some strange reason, they could not understand what I was desperately trying to say to them. I liked them very much, and, they seemed to like me. In fact, my older brother Ricky, almost every night before I went to bed, would read a poem to me that he wrote himself. Boy, I loved those words:

"Babies come in many sizes—chubby, long or small.
My brother's 7lb. 3oz. and 19" tall.
We begged mom for years to have a child, and finally he's here.
He looks up at me when in my arms and doesn't shed a tear.
I help change his diapers when he's wet, and burp him when he's fed,
And I make sure to get a goodnight kiss before I go to bed.
I read him stories when I can, I'm sure he understands.
We'll have so many things to do, I have so many plans!
We'll ride our bikes, we'll play football, and I'll buy him a ball to throw,
But I can't do too much with him right now, looks like he'll have to grow!
For now I'll keep him safe from harm, and watch him as he grows,

For he's also growing deep within my heart as I hold him, nice and close!"

Boy, what a family! Mommy and daddy really raised them well! I really love my family, and they seem to love me!

2 YEARS OLD

I am now two years old, and, for the past several months, mommy has been looking very strange, just as if someone were blowing her up just like a balloon. She just keeps getting bigger and bigger! Then, just when it looked like she was ready to pop, she disappeared. I don't know where she went. I haven't seen her for a few days. No one else seems worried, so I guess she hasn't exploded yet. I have seen it happen to too many of my balloons, and I don't want my mommy to burst. Then, daddy picks me up in those strong arms of his, gives me a big hug, and says, "Anthony, your mommy is having another baby!" I don't quite understand what that means until daddy comes home that afternoon with mommy. As he helps her out of the car, I notice that her belly is not big anymore! Plus, I notice that she's holding something pink in her arms, wrapped in a blue blanket. Daddy says that this little pink bundle in the blue blanket is my little brother Andrew Marcus. He is no longer resting in mommy's belly. This is great! Not only is mommy OK, but she has also brought home a nice, soft new toy for me to play with! Mommy and daddy caution me that I can look at him, but I can't play with him, not just yet. That's when I realize that, Andy is not MY toy, he is THEIR toy! They say that I can play with him when I get older, but I hope they don't break him before I get a chance to play with him!

3 YEARS OLD

Now three years old, I am beginning to feel more like an adult, more like my brothers and sisters. I am very curious, and insist on learning all there is to know about everything and everyone. Sometimes when I say something, my brothers or sisters will say, "Who taught him that?" or "How did he learn that?", or "He's talking very well!" Why not, I wonder! Give me credit for some intelligence! After all, I am an adult just like you! Also, I have got so much energy! I can run all over the house, jump from every piece of furniture in the house, hang from the chandelier, interrupt everything my brothers and sisters are doing, and STILL have enough energy to "help" my mommy and daddy with whatever they are doing. For the longest time, everyone was telling me to speak, and they couldn't wait for me to take my first step. They just couldn't wait until I started walking and talking. Now, all I hear is "Tony, will you *please* sit down and shut up!" I sure wish that they would make up their minds!

3

Childhood Firsts

MY FIRST SNOW!

It was a chilly, wintry morning in December 1959. I was now 6 years old. Mommy had promised me that this year I could go out in the snow to play with my brothers and sisters. I had been waiting for months but, so far, not one single snowflake! Now, as I slowly rose from sleep, I could feel the icy chill that had settled in the air just above my blanket. As I gradually sat up, rubbing the sleep from my eyes, I noticed that my room was brighter than usual this morning. I jumped out of bed, ran to the window, and just stared—stared at the glistening white snow that seemed to fill the world outside! Beautiful, heavenly white snow EVERYWHERE—on the rooftops, in the trees, on the cars, on the streets, everywhere, as far as the eyes could see!! I fairly danced around the room with excitement, not even noticing how cold the bedroom floor was on my bare feet! "Mommy! Mommy! It snowed, it snowed!!" I shouted. So, while mommy was busy preparing breakfast for the family, daddy helped me to get washed up and to find clothes to put on. When I was washed and dressed, I rushed down the stairs to eat breakfast. I ate breakfast in record time this morning, and then asked to be excused from the table. Then, mommy proceeded to turn her six-year old son into the abominable snowman—coat, hat, scarf, leggings, long underwear, boots, the works. Finally, she said, "All done"! She opened the front door for me, and I rushed outside to play and have fun in my first snow!

Brother, Ricky, Jackie and Mary Ann were already outside, running and playing in the still falling snow. I stood there for a few minutes, in my new, glistening white world, wondering what I should do first. Suddenly, a huge snowball came sailing just INCHES past my head! I quickly turned to see my brother Ricky, running and laughing at how close he had come to bouncing a snowball off the top of my head! Soon, other kids joined in the fun, snowballs and uncontrollable laughter filling the air! School, food, chores—ALL were forgotten! There were so many fun and exciting things to do in the glorious white snow! It was great fun to run up to the top of the hill with huge pieces of cardboard. Then, once at the top, we would sit on the cardboard, grab the sides, and GO! We would sail down the hill at 100 miles an hour, legs sticking straight up in the air!! When we tired of this, we would fall into the snow and wave our arms up and down, making angels in the fallen snow. We would build snow barricades and have huge snowball battles. We would just roll around in the snow, laughing and shouting! It was great! Everyone was having fun outside, and everyone was laughing. This had been the best day of my young life, and I didn't want it to end.

Sadly though, the fun ended all too quickly, as mothers called their soaking wet but happy children in for dinner. Then, after dinner, tired little children slowly drifted off to sleep, dreaming of fun-filled times in today's "wonderful world of snow"! Mommy helped me to undress and prepare to take a bath, and then she dressed me warmly for bed. Later, daddy quietly tiptoed into my room and tucked me in, making sure that I was nice and warm as, once again, I slowly drifted off to sleep.

I remember a few years later my father bought wooden sleds for us. They were great! We would swiftly eat breakfast, throw on our outdoor clothes, all 20 pounds of it, and race to the baseball field near our home. There was a long hill there, just PERFECT for sled riding! We would start at the top of the hill on level ground, run with our sled, and hop on just before going down the hill. Doing it this way, we could go down the hill at great speed. One time, as I was going down the hill, my sled hit a large rock hidden beneath the snow. My sled stopped, but I didn't! My body kept going, my left hand got twisted up underneath me, and I fractured my wrist. My parents rushed me to the hospital, and stayed with me while my wrist was set, and a cast was put on. My father didn't holler at me, but carefully took the time to explain to me and my brothers and sisters how to carefully, and safely, ride a sled.

MY FIRST FISHING TRIP

At seven years of age, my parents decided that it was time to take me on my first fishing trip. Mommy loved to fish, so she and daddy would often go on fishing trips together. Today, they decided to take the children along. So, we all piled into the station wagon, and headed out for what was to be my first (and last!) fishing trip. We traveled for several hours, and, after many choruses of "Are we there yet?" and numerous stops for bathroom breaks, we finally arrived at our destination. I got out of the car and stretched. I had been squished between Brother and Ricky the whole trip, and it was great to be finally able to move again. After stretching again, I decided to look around to see where we were. I was fascinated by what I saw! We were at a beautiful, strikingly clear blue lake, surrounded by tall, majestic pine trees. Pine needles were scattered all over the ground underneath these trees. The air was so fresh and clean, that it felt great to take long deep breaths. Brightly colored birds were singing and fluttering about high in the trees. Ducks of various sizes and colors were swimming on the lake, and you could walk right up to them on concrete pathways that led right into the lake. I could also see boats of various sizes already on the lake, filled with fishermen, lines already cast into the water, anxiously awaiting that first bite. While my family got the fishing gear out of the car, I decided that it was just too beautiful to stand there and do nothing. Everything, to me, was just breath taking.

I started walking along one of the pathways to the lake. I couldn't keep my eyes off of the ducks gliding gracefully through the water, every so often dipping their heads elegantly into the water for a nice, cool drink. I stopped for a moment, kneeling down to get a closer look at one of the ducks. "Be careful!" my brother cried out, "There are crayfish in there!" Startled, I quickly turned towards my brother to ask him what in the world a crayfish was. Boy, was that the wrong thing to do! I slipped, lost my balance, and fell into the water! "Help me, help me!" I screamed, my eyes searching the water frantically for those giant, killer crayfish my brother had tried to warn me about. The water wasn't very deep where I fell in and, had I just stood up, the water probably would have been just above my waist. But, I was too busy trying not to get eaten alive to notice! My father came running towards me, and I was still close enough to the walkway for my father to just reach out and grab hold of my shirt. He pulled me toward him, and then up out of the water. "Anthony, are you all right?" he asked. I was cold, scared and soaking wet, but I was all right! For some reason, the crayfish had decided not to attack me. My father carried me back to the car where, for me, things went from bad to worse. I was still soaking wet, and my parents had not brought any spare clothes for me. My mother had placed a few of my sister's dresses in the car to take to the cleaners, so I had to get out of my wet clothes, and slowly put on one of my sister's dresses.

It was humiliating! I had to wear that dress for the remainder of our fishing trip, and then all the way home. Once we arrived home, I had to run from the car to the house, but not before some of my friends had seen me in my sister's dress! For weeks, I had to endure the teasing of my friends, including being called Antoinette! At school I was asked if I had shoes and a matching purse for that dress. Someone even brought in earrings for me to wear! They said that it had taken a while to find just the right earrings, but they were sure that they would match my dress! This was an experience I will never forget, and I have never gone fishing since!

MY FIRST SWIMMING LESSON

My father was a member of the U.S. Army Reserve, and he was sometimes stationed at an army base at Sandusky, Ohio. Part of the Base was located right on the beaches of Lake Erie. I can remember that there was a movie theatre on the Base, and admission was very cheap. There was also a small store where we could buy candy, chips, cookies, sodas, and other "necessities of life". The store also had a section where we could play video games. I remember getting up one morning, getting dressed, eating, and heading towards the door with Andy. "Be careful where you two step", mommy cried as we went outside to look for Ricky and Mary Ann. As we began to walk outside, we heard, and felt under our feet, a lot of crunching noises. We glanced down, and noticed that the sidewalk was filled with bugs! We were told that they were called "soldiers", but we sure didn't want any part of them.

It was here that I had my first swimming lesson. I was eight years old, and I was very nervous. As I sat on the edge of the army cot in my room, slowly putting on my trunks, my life flashed before my eyes (several times, for it was a very short life!) I really didn't want to do this! "Come on, Tony" Dad said, "You will be just fine". Slowly, I walked out of the room with my father, and out onto the beach. All I could see was sparkling blue water—nothing but water for miles and miles! Dad took my hand, and we slowly walked into the water, the wet sand squishing between my toes. I walked very carefully, so as not to step on a seashell or some other strange sea creature. Together, we waded in until the water was just up to my chest. Then, my father said "Wait right there, Tony." Dad waded out a few feet farther, turned around and said, "OK Tony, swim towards me. Close your eyes, stretch out, and paddle towards me with your arms and legs, just like I showed you." So, I closed my eyes, stretched out, and paddled frantically for what seemed like hours. Then, I opened my eyes, and sure enough, there was my father, standing right in front of me. "I did it! I did it!" I shouted! "Yes you did just fine, my son." my father replied. "Now, let's practice just a little bit longer." So, for about another hour or so, I practiced swimming with my father. It was always fun when we could spend time together, just him and I. I found out later, though, that I had not really been swimming. As soon as I had closed my eyes, my father had hurriedly moved towards me, trying to build my confidence in my own ability to swim. He firmly believed that, if I had enough confidence in myself, I could do just about anything! Oddly enough, I began to believe it also. This is one lesson that I have never forgotten! It has carried me through life. I learned to have confidence in myself, and in what I could do. I have achieved a modicum of success in every endeavor, for, just as my father taught me, I firmly believed that I could do just about anything I set my mind to do.

MY FIRST LOVE

I was only nine years old when I first saw her. Just one look was all it took! I fell madly, deeply in love (well, as deeply in love as a nine year old boy could get!) At the time, my father was a mechanical engineer for one of the local hospitals. A woman he worked with, Mrs. Oakes, needed someone to baby-sit her two children—an eight-year-old girl, and a six-year-old boy. My father said that he would speak to his daughter Mary Ann, to see if she was able to do it. So, he spoke with my sister Mary Ann that evening, and she gladly accepted the babysitting job. After the first few days, Mrs. Oakes saw that she got along well with Mary Ann, and so did her children. After babysitting for several weeks, Mary Ann said to me "Tony, the little girl I am babysitting is very pretty! Mrs. Oakes said that I could bring her and her little brother over to our house tomorrow to meet our family." Well, I was so nervous that night that I could hardly get to sleep! I woke up very early the next morning, washed, put on my best clothes, put on some of my older brother's cologne, and sat at my sister's bedroom window waiting to get my first glimpse of that "pretty girl!" Finally, I noticed Mary Ann walking up the street, with a child holding onto each hand.

As they got closer, I could see the little girl. Boy, was my sister wrong! That little girl wasn't pretty, she was beautiful! She wasn't very tall, but she had long, silky dark hair, beautiful almond shaped brown eyes, and an enchanting smile that could make me forget my own name every time she glanced at me, or whenever I even thought of her! I fell in love instantly, but, being shy, I had no idea what to say to her. My family had a lot of fun with this. For example, my oldest brother, knowing that I had a crush on her, would pick her up and run around the yard with her, with me chasing closely behind him. I had to rescue my sweetheart, and thus to her how much I loved her. I didn't realize then just how ridiculous this was, but my brothers really had fun with this. Every time we chose sides for dodge ball with our friends, and she wound up on the opposite team, I would refuse to throw the ball at her, despite the angry shouts of my team members. How could I possibly hit the woman I love?

I treasured every moment I could spend with her, but I just couldn't tell her. Every time I tried to speak with her, the only words that would come out of my mouth were "yes" or "no". I felt very foolish, but my extreme shyness was preventing me from expressing my true feelings. I realized that, if I wasn't able to tell her how I felt, I just might lose her. I decided to write her a poem, expressing my true feelings. So, I spent the next few days in my room, trying desperately to put my feelings into words. Finally, I was finished. The poem that would tell my new found "girl friend" how I really felt about her was finished. I called it "LOVE":

Love is something none can see,
a feeling in your heart.
This feeling makes you sad the day
the one you love must part.
It's there when you are holding hands,
and when you walk together.
When you sit and think of the one you love,
THOSE thoughts are what you treasure.
Perhaps there's more to love than this,
perhaps it's something real.

For whenever I see you or hear your voice,
I KNOW it's love I feel.
What I hope for most of all, for you, dear one, and me,
   is to get married and live in happiness, perhaps eternally!!

Next, I had to carefully plan how to give my poem to her. I would wait until just the right moment, walk up to her, look her right in those big, beautiful brown eyes, and say, "Shirley Anne, I wrote this poem just for you. It says just how deeply I care about you." Yes, my plan was perfect! My chance came the very next day. My sister brought Shirley Anne over to our house, and the three of us sat in the living room together watching television. Finally, Mary Ann left the room. She told Shirley that she was going to the kitchen to get something to eat. This was the perfect opportunity! I slowly stood up, and took the poem out of my pocket. Then, without saying a word, and without thinking, I threw the poem at Shirley and then quickly ran out of the room! No, No! That was not the way I had planned it! Humiliated, I didn't think I could ever face her again. I just stood in the kitchen with my head down, staring at my shoes. I wished that I could just disappear off the face of the earth! Then, I heard someone walking towards me. Slowly, I raised my head, and found myself face to face with Shirley Anne. I just stood there, motionless, like a deer frozen in the headlights of an oncoming car. What should I do?? What could I possibly say to her? She stood there for a moment, and then she smiled at me. Then, she said, "Tony, that was a beautiful poem! Thank you very much!" Well, she didn't think me a fool after all! Who knows, in time she may even get to like me! I sincerely hoped so, for she was a very special girl.

A few weeks later, Mary Ann was taking Shirley to the movies to see *The Incredible Journey* and asked if I wanted to come. What a foolish question! I put on my best play clothes, and again borrowed some of my brother's cologne. When Mary Ann was ready, I hopped in the back seat of her car. I reserved the front seat for that special person. We then drove to Shirley's house and blew the horn. The vision of loveliness came out of the house, and all I could do was stare as she opened the front door. She walked down the steps (I could almost swear that her feet did not touch the steps), said hello to Mary Ann and I, hopped in the front seat, and gracefully put her seat belt on. I sat in the back seat speechless, as Mary Ann and Shirley chatted. When we arrived at the theatre, Shirley said, "Tony, would you like an ice cream sandwich?" I looked at Mary Ann, and she nodded her head to let me know that it would be all right. So, I replied, "Yes, thank you." Shirley bought the ice cream, Mary Ann bought the tickets, and I watched Shirley. We walked in, found our seats, and anxiously awaited the start of the movie. Shirley and my sister Mary Ann really enjoyed the movie. I enjoyed the ice cream my true love had purchased for me, and I enjoyed just being in her company.

As Shirley and her brother grew older, they no longer needed a sitter. Mary Ann retired from the babysitting business, so I saw Shirley on and off after that. I just couldn't get her out of my mind. She went to Wilkinsburg High School, and I attended Central Catholic High School. I got out earlier than she did, so I decided to meet her after school and walk her home. I was very shy, so, for the entire walk home, I didn't say a word. Shirley would try to start a conversation, but my responses would be very brief, a "yes" or a "no" answer, and that was about it. I would walk her to her front door, say "goodbye", and then walk home. Actually, I would drift home, on cloud nine. When I was bold enough, I decided to start walking to see her at her home. So, several days a week, I would walk to her house, listening to music on my radio along the way. When I reached her home, I would knock on the door. When the door opened, I would say hello to Mrs. Oakes, and hello to the girl that I loved. They would invite me in, and I would sit down and watch TV with her, or help her with her homework. I never said much, and since I always had difficulty saying goodbye, I would be there pretty late. In fact, on Saturday nights, I would be there until Chiller Theatre went off, and Chillie Billie Cardille said goodnight. Shirley would turn off the TV, I would say goodnight, and walk home.

I also remember the time when I had fractured my ankle, and I was on crutches. My mom came home and told me that she had met Shirley and her mom at the grocery store, and told them about my ankle. My mom had said to Shirley that it might be a good idea to stop by and see Tony. When my mom arrived home and told me this, I quickly hopped up the stairs, washed my face, brushed my teeth, combed my hair, and put on some of my own cologne, Jovan Musk. I hopped into my room and put on my best gray pants and burgundy shirt. Then, I hopped back downstairs, sat on the couch, and continued working on a poster that I was doing for school on the effects of drinking and smoking. When Shirley arrived, my mom let her in, and she said, "Hello, Tony. What happened to you?" So, we talked for a while, and she commented on how good my poster was. I realized, then and there, that this was someone that I wanted to spend the rest of my life with. So, I spent a lot of time with her after that. I was determined to date her as often and as long as possible to get her to like me.

When I graduated from Central Catholic High School, Shirley and her mom gave me a graduation gift—a beautiful, very expensive-looking wristwatch. I loved it! I received offers from Michigan State, West Point, and Notre Dame to attend college, and I was listed in "Who's Who Among American High School Students". I decided to rest a year before going to college, and, in that year, something happened. At 18 years of age, I decided to propose. I asked Shirley to accompany me to a jewelry store downtown, supposedly to get my watch fixed. When we got there, I told Shirley that I loved her, and wanted to marry her. I told her that she could pick out her engagement ring and our wedding bands. The real reason for our visit to the jewelry store was for me to propose, not to get a watch repaired. She was excited, but said that she would prefer to get her rings at a better quality jewelry store in Monroeville Mall. So, we drove to the Mall, and selected our rings. We were now officially engaged, and on December 16, 1972 we became Mr. and Mrs. Luck. I went to college many years later, and I have never regretted getting married.

In my opinion, though, 19 years of age is too early for someone to get married. I would never recommend to anyone to get married at such an early age. You need to have more experience in life, experience that will make you more mature, and thus a better marriage mate. You will also know and understand yourself better. This will help you to have a better and more successful marriage. For us, we made a lot of mistakes that we may not have made had we been older when we got married. Nevertheless, I married the girl of my dreams, and I was happy!

MY FIRST FIRECRACKER!

We lived in a pretty big home due to the size of our family. Starting downstairs, we had a finished basement with ½ a bath, bar, pool table and ping-pong table. I can remember my sisters Jackie and Mary Ann having dance parties down there with their friends.

On the first floor, we had a large living room, a nice-sized dining room, and a full-sized kitchen. In the dining room, we had a large chest freezer with a lock. Every Halloween, my parents would place all of the candy that we had collected in there. They would then give out this candy to us a little at a time, so that we would not get sick. I remember them telling us that if you eat too much candy, you can get worms, or your teeth can fall out. My father always took us different places for Halloween, so we always got a lot of candy! In one neighborhood, we were given hot dogs and hamburgers instead of candy. It was great! It was a lot of fun when our father was able to spend time with us, for we loved him. The only bad part of Halloween was the dreaded Cod Liver Oil my mother would spoon-feed us after we ate the candy.

We had a full front porch that went the whole length of the front of the house. The house roof also covered it, and one side was enclosed. We had a small back porch, a yard that went completely around the house, and a large, detached two-car garage. In the back yard, we had a "Tarzan" swing in one of the huge weeping willow trees. It was nothing more than a thick rope with a big knot tied on the end. We would run up the walk, grab the swing, and swing back and forth. One time, my hands slipped while the swing was going up. I landed with a thud on the concrete walk, ½ of my face on the concrete, ½ in the dirt. My eyeglasses broke, and I felt dizzy. I stumbled into the house and fell onto the couch in the living room. My father came in and said, "Tony, what's wrong?" I mumbled, "I'm OK." My father took one look at me, and then picked up my glasses and looked at them. He knew something was wrong. He said, "Let's go, Tony" and he took me to the hospital emergency room. I was OK, just badly bruised.

On the second floor we had four bedrooms and a bathroom. My mom and dad shared one room, my two older brothers shared a room, my two older sisters shared a room, and my three younger sisters shared a room.

The third floor was a finished attic the length of the house, with a lower ceiling and walk-in closet. This is where my younger brother Andy and I slept.

It was a neighborhood tradition at that time for young people to stand around in the evening with their friends, telling jokes or scary stories. I was around twelve years old, and I was standing in front of our home one evening with my brothers Ricky and Andy, and some of our friends. We were telling jokes and swapping stories, when the subject of firecrackers came up. It was illegal to purchase or use firecrackers where we lived, but one of our friends said that he knew how to make them at home. A hush fell over us as, full of curiosity, we asked him "How?" He explained, excited that he had everyone's undivided attention. That evening, I just couldn't stop thinking, "Homemade firecrackers! What a great idea!"

So, the next day, I took the things we had talked about the night before, and ran up to my attic bedroom to make my first firecracker. When I was finished, it didn't look much like a firecracker. I lit it, covered my ears, closed my eyes, and KABOOM, it worked! There were little bits of fire all over the room, including a pair of my brother Andy's underwear! My excitement turned to horror when I noticed that his underwear were on fire! Alarmed, I quickly stamped the fire out with my shoe, and threw Andy's underwear under some clothes in the closet. "He will never know what happened!" I thought. Of course, being young at the time, I didn't realize that clothing still smolders even after the fire has been put out. Soon, smoke started pouring out of the closet! Panic-stricken, I opened the attic window to let out the smoke. Another bad idea, because that let in more oxygen to feed the fire, making it worse! The smoke started to fill the bedroom, and it was billowing out the window. Now what do I do? What do I do? Then, an idea came to me! I will just lie on my bed and pretend to be asleep! Hopefully, someone will come up to get me, and I will pretend that I have no idea how the fire started. I heard someone running up the steps, so I quickly lay down and started snoring. "Tony, Tony, wake up, the house is on fire!!" screamed Ricky! "What? I jumped up, still pretending to be a little groggy from sleep. "Oh no, I could have died!" I said. He told me as we ran down the stairs, that one of our neighbors had seen the smoke pouring out of the attic window, and had called the fire department. We ran down the stairs and joined the rest of the family outside.

When it was all over, we all just stood there in total disbelief, staring at what once was our beautiful home! Since the fire started in the attic, the firemen had to cut holes in the roof to put the fire out. We had water and smoke damage on all three floors of our home. Everything was ruined! My father and mother had to contact several United Way organizations, and they assisted us in getting food, clothing, and a temporary place to live. I remember going with my brothers and sisters to shoe stores, looking for shoes to wear. We went to second hand stores, trying to find economical clothing for each member of my family. Arrangements were made for us to visit food banks and other organizations to get food for the family. Arrangements were then made for our family to move temporarily into a vacant house across the street while our home was being repaired. The firemen explained to my parents that the cause of the fire was probably faulty electrical wiring in the attic closet, so it looked like I was off the hook. No one would ever know that I had started the fire! So, we spent the holidays in a borrowed home, wearing borrowed clothes, eating borrowed food, all because of me!

I remember my father getting a huge tree for Christmas. He always managed to get a tree big enough to touch the ceiling. He placed the base of the tree in a metal tree holder, and filled the holder with sugar water, so that the tree would last a few days longer. Then, we had the fun of decorating it as a family. That night, I couldn't get to sleep thinking about what I had done, so, I went downstairs to look at the tree. I tried to get under it to see if there was enough sugar water, and the tree fell over on top of me! Afraid of causing yet another problem for my family, and my father, I frantically fought with the tree, desperately trying to get it back up again before someone else came downstairs. I didn't have my pajama top on, just the bottoms, so the pine needles made nice little scratches on my chest and arms. Finally, I got it upright again. I made sure that the decorations were all intact, and refilled the sugar water in the base. I cleaned up as best I could, and wearily, I went back to bed.

Years later, after my father had died, I found out from a friend of the family that, when the fire happened, my father had actually cried! He just sat there, shaking his head, repeating over and over again, "What am I going to do?" He had lost his home, his possessions, everything, and it was just weeks before the Christmas holidays! He had a wife and nine children, with absolutely no place to live, and it was all my fault! I didn't know at the time all the pain and suffering I had caused my father, and my family, all because of a homemade firecracker. It is too late now to tell my father how very sorry I am, for he is gone. What I do know is that I had set the house on fire, caused all of that damage, all of that suffering, and then LIED about it! Dad, mom, brothers and sisters, I am very, very sorry! I never meant to set fire to our home, and cause so much pain and suffering for my parents and my family. I love my parents, and I love my family. Looking back, I should NEVER have made that firecracker. I should never have set our house on fire, and I will never, ever, tell a lie again!

MY FIRST JOB

At 12 years of age, my brother Andy and I accepted our first job, delivering food circulars for the local grocery store. We delivered circulars once a week, and we were paid $3.00 each. Since candy bars were just 5 cents each, $3.00 was a lot of money! Plus, we got to be friends with the grocery store owner and his family. We also got to know our neighbors a little better, especially the ones who called and complained that they didn't get their circulars! I remember daddy telling us how important it was that the circulars be neatly rolled and tied with a rubber band. We also had to make sure that every circular fell neatly on a porch, not in the yard or in bushes. He also helped me to see, as I took on grass cutting and other jobs in the next few years, how important it is to always give 100%. My father told us that, when you agree to do a job or to perform a service, make sure you give what you agreed to give, and do your job to the best of your ability.

I remember one grass-cutting job in particular. I slipped while I was cutting the grass, and my foot went underneath the power mower. The blades cut off the top of my tennis shoe, along with part of my sock. I stopped the mower, and cautiously looked down at my foot, expecting to see blood gushing out of my tennis shoe, and my toes scattered all over the lawn. Thankfully, all of my toes were intact! I had pulled my foot away just before the lawnmower blades had gotten to my toes. When my father came to pick me up, he was shocked when he saw the lawn. I had the blades of the lawn mower set too low, and the lawn looked terrible. There were bald patches everywhere! My father had to straighten it out with the owners. He never hollered at me about my tennis shoe or about the lawn. He was grateful that my toes were still there, and he explained to me how important it was to always check the settings on the lawnmower before cutting the grass.

My father and my sister Mary Ann were instrumental in helping me to get my first job. I accepted my first real job at age 16. I was a stock boy at G. C. Murphy & Co. I remembered everything my father had taught me, and the manager was glad he hired me. When someone on the sales floor needed supplies, they called me in the stockroom, and I would bring them down. If the restaurant drink station ran low, I was called to replace the syrup tanks. If there was a spill on the sales floor, I was called to clean it up. If someone made a mess in the restrooms, I was called to clean it up. I didn't enjoy cleaning toilets, but my father had taught me always to give 100%. So, even when cleaning toilets, I gave 100%, to the best of my ability. My father was always able to find employment for us through his contacts. He made friends easily, and he had a lot of friends.

MY FIRST MUSICAL GROUP

My parents paid for music lessons for us, and my brothers Ricky, Andy and I learned to play the drums. In grade school, I played the big bass drum. As he got older, my parents purchased a drum set for my brother Ricky, and he played for a while. When he stopped, I began to play. I loved it, so I decided to get a band together. At first, I had a bass guitar, a lead guitar, and myself. We practiced on my porch, and I thought it sounded great. One of my younger sisters was having a dance party in the basement, so I asked her if we could come down and play for them. She said yes, and I ran upstairs to tell the group. We had our first engagement! We carried all of our equipment downstairs, set up, and started playing. A few minutes later, after the complaints of her friends, my sister asked if we could stop and go back upstairs. We were humiliated! A group of young children had told us that we "stink"! I decided, then and there, that I would never again subject my group to another experience like that. We would practice in earnest, every day if possible, until we were really good. Then, we would practice some more. Later, I added a conga drummer, a keyboard player, and two singers to the group. We played at wedding receptions, parties, and once at the Typographical Hall in downtown Pittsburgh. There was nothing better than watching people dancing, and having fun, listening to the music that we were creating. I decided to have my group play at my own wedding. I had to leave the group, because it took too much time to practice and also be a husband, so they had another drummer perform. I have only played several times since I have been married, and I miss it. Perhaps, one day I will buy another drum set, and play in my garage where it won't upset the neighbors.

4

Memories Of Daddy Today

Reflecting back on the years of growing up with my father, I try to remember all of the things he did for me. I remember how, at 16 years of age, he taught me how to drive. I remember when he took me to the State Police Barracks for my driver's test. I did great on the questions. The driving test was fine, until I tried to turn the family station wagon around in that narrow turnaround. I failed twice, and finally passed the third time. Each time, I received encouragement and support from my parents. Then, I was permitted to use the family station wagon whenever I wanted to. My parents trusted me, and gave me a lot of freedom. I remember when, at 17 years of age, I had to make a decision on which religion to follow. My father, though he did not agree with my decision, was still there for me whenever I needed him. Then, at 19 years of age, I decided to get married to Shirley Anne, the girl that I met when I was nine years old. My father was there at our wedding and at our reception. Throughout our married lives, whenever we needed him, he was there. When we moved into our first home, my dad was there to provide encouragement and support. He told us what we needed to do to set a good example for the community—how to take care of the lawn, the shrubs, etc.

Today, I am 48 years old, and Shirley Anne and I have four children—Stacey Leigh, Peter Alexander, Stephen Anthony, and Nicholas Ian. My son Peter met and married a young woman who my wife and I have also grown to love. Her name is Monique. I try to share with my children the same wisdom, knowledge and love my father shared with me. I try to be there for them just as my father was there for me. With a family of my own now, it becomes easier to reflect back on life experiences, and realize that my mom and dad loved us so very much. My mom now lives in South Carolina. I don't see her very much, but we try to keep in touch with cards, letters, phone calls and e-mail.

I can remember the fun times we had as a family. Every year, my father would take us to West View Park, Kennywood Park, or Cedar Point Park. My father also enjoyed taking us to the Allegheny County Fairs. At the Fairs, we got to see farm animals, farm machinery, and learn how people in rural America live and work. One year we met the comedians Martin and Rossi, and saw the Banana Splits in person. I remember that, it was only at these times of the year that my father could relax and spend time with his family. These were the times that we could really get to know our father. He was always so busy the remainder of the year working three or four jobs, struggling to support his family. At this one time of the year, he would play with us, ride with us, eat with us, and spend time with us. We really enjoyed his company! My dad always brought along with us his motion picture camera so that he could record our family events for the future. My mom still has those old movies. Whenever we watch them, it is easy to see how much our father loved us! We can see ourselves when we were small children, riding in KiddieLand, having a great time, while my father was taking pictures. We watch as we slide down snow-covered hills on our cardboard. We watch as my father enjoys having fun with his family.

I can also remember my father's times of instruction, where he tried to prepare us for life ahead. Some of the favorite phrases he used to teach us were:

- "Be grateful for what you have. It beats a blank."

- "There is no such thing as can't"

- "Believe in yourself, and you can accomplish anything."

- "There is no-one better than you, and you are no better than anyone else."

Through the years, my dad was always there when we needed him. Whenever I had marital questions, he was there with the answers. When I needed employment, he always knew the right people to contact to find me a good job. He was always courteous, and treated people the way that he wanted to be treated, so he was very popular, and had a lot of friends. Even when my wife and I moved into our first home, my father was there with advice and assistance.

I can remember also the times when I caused my father pain and sorrow. As a young teenager, I remember getting upset with dad because he didn't have the money to provide what I thought was the right gift for a birthday party I had been invited to. How foolish! How could I get upset with a loving father who was holding down four jobs trying to support a wife and eight children! I just didn't understand.

My mother would deep-fry chicken, and I remember one time I tiptoed into the kitchen when I thought no one was watching me. I turned on the kitchen faucet, put my hand under the water, and started sprinkling water into the pan of grease with my fingers.

The water would make the hot grease dance and bubble, and it was fun to watch. Fun, that is, until I heard my father's voice say, "What are you doing?" Surprised, I said, "Nothing!" My father twisted my arm behind my back, and asked again what I was doing. I told him exactly what I was doing, in great detail. As a matter of fact, I was willing to tell him anything else he wanted to know about me or any of my brothers or sisters at this point! He released my arm, and told me to go up to my room. I didn't realize it then, but my father was really worried about me. I could have been seriously burned, or otherwise injured myself or someone else if I continued to do that. I also could have started another fire! I never did that again, though. With a family of my own, I understand now, but it's too late to tell him, to thank him.

I remember the last time that I saw my father alive and well. He was visiting Pittsburgh, and decided to make a surprise visit to see me at work. When my supervisor called me over to her desk and said that my father was down in the public office to see me, I just couldn't believe it! I fairly flew down the steps to the Public Office! My father, when he noticed me, started walking towards me, smiling, with his hand out-stretched. I ignored his hand, grabbed him and said, "Give me a hug!" He introduced me to his new wife, and we talked for a while. I did not know at the time that this would be the last hug I would ever receive from my dad. This would be the last time I would be able to hold him, or tell him how much I love him. I would not see him again until he was in the hospital, unconscious, his life slowly slipping away. I just stood there, motionless, helpless, as my father's life slowly came to an end. My father is gone now, but he will never be forgotten. His family, his friends, and most of all, his son, will always remember his kindness, his warmth, and his love! He lives on in our memories, and he lives on through the pages of this book. I look forward to the day when I can once again put my arms around him and say, "I love you daddy!" I will always love you daddy, and I long for the day when, hopefully, I will see you again. Farewell, daddy. I miss you very much!

5

The Final Chapter?

The Bible, at Ecclesiastes 9:11 tells us, in part, that "the swift do not have the race, nor the mighty ones the battle…because time and unforeseen occurrence befall them all." These prophetic words rang true for me on May 6, 1999, the day that I was diagnosed with the same cancer that took the life of my father—Multiple Myeloma! Several months prior to May 6, my health began to take a noticeable turn for the worst. I began experiencing difficulty going up steps, and I couldn't walk for any distance without stopping to catch my breath. I seemed to get winded very easily. I also kept catching colds and, at one point, I even developed pneumonia. I also experienced nosebleeds, something I had never experienced before. My nose would bleed for several hours at a time. It didn't matter how I positioned my head, or what I used on my nose, I couldn't get the bleeding to stop. I also developed tiny, itchy red blotches all over my face, hands, arms, and legs, even the soles of my feet. So, I made an appointment with my Primary Care Physician for a complete checkup. He performed a complete physical examination, ran some tests, and did some blood work. After the examination, the doctor told me that the nosebleeds were probably due to dry heat in my home. The difficulty going up steps, he said, was probably due to anemia. He said I would receive a call from his office if the blood work showed anything out of the ordinary. He also referred me to a dermatologist for the red blotches.

To my surprise, when we returned home, there was a voice mail message from my doctor—not a nurse, or a secretary, but the doctor himself! The message was that it is important that I contact his office.

So, I contacted his office, and made an appointment to see him the next day. When I arrived, my doctor wasn't in, but they said that another doctor would see me. They had me sit in one of those smaller rooms, on a table covered with white "wrapping paper", waiting for the doctor to come in. About five minutes later, the doctor came in, and started explaining something to me in medical terms that I did not understand. I stopped him and said, "Could you please explain what's wrong with me in English?" He replied, "After reviewing the results of your blood work, we are going to refer you to a Hematologist/Oncologist, because it appears that you may have a form of blood cancer". I just sat there, numb. I couldn't say anything. He held out a card for me, with the name and number of the Hematologist/Oncologist he was referring me to. I took it, stood up, and walked out of the office, and into my car. I went home, and immediately called the number the doctor gave me. To my dismay, the voice on the other end said that the first available appointment for the doctor I had been referred to was over a month away. Angrily, I said, "This is urgent! I am willing to see ANY Hematologist/Oncologist there!" So, they gave me an appointment with another Hematologist/Oncologist in the practice for the following week, May 6 at 1pm.

I also made an appointment with the Dermatologist. When I went into her office, she asked me to take off my clothes and put on a hospital gown. Then, she looked closely at the red blotches that covered my body. She closely examined my arms and legs. Because she couldn't tell precisely what it was or what was causing it, she said that she wanted to perform a biopsy on my arms. I agreed, and she took a sample of skin from each arm. She then applied bandages to both arms and said I would receive a call when she had the results. Her diagnosis? The red blotches were actually eczema, or extremely dry skin. She gave me a prescription for a cream that I could apply on my skin to alleviate the itching. So, the rash turned out to be something that was not too serious, something that I could live with. I hoped that my appointment with the Oncologist would work out the same way.

Thus, on May 6, 1999, I went to work as usual. I was working at a new career, and I was just beginning month six of my six-month probation period. I decided to go to the Oncologist during my lunch hour to find out what was going on. When I arrived at her office, she took me right in. She asked me if I ever had a blood transfusion, and I said no. I thought to myself, what disease could I possibly have that she thinks I got from a blood transfusion? She then asked if I would be averse to having a blood transfusion. I replied, "I am sorry. I will not accept a blood transfusion." She asked, "So you would rather die?" I replied, "No, I do NOT wish to die. I am willing to accept whatever treatments you recommend, and take whatever medication you prescribe. You know a lot more about this than I do. I am just not willing to accept a blood transfusion. What, may I ask, is going on? What is wrong with me?" The Oncologist replied that I might have Multiple Myeloma, a form of bone cancer. Her pager went off, so she excused herself, and left the room for a few minutes. I just sat there, motionless, desperately trying to hold back the tears, wondering, "What does this mean?" Questions raced through my mind—Is she serious? Why is this happening to me? Am I going to die? What about my wife and children? What type of cancer was that? Can she cure it? I was afraid to ask those questions, because I was afraid to hear the answers. She returned to the room, and asked if I would be willing to admit myself into the hospital today, to get a biopsy done to confirm her diagnosis. A biopsy? What in the world does that mean? At the time, I didn't know what that meant, and I didn't want to know. I informed the Oncologist that I would admit myself that afternoon. I thanked her, and left the office. I drove slowly back to work, driving from memory because my eyes just stared straight ahead in shock and disbelief.

When I arrived at work, I went into my office, and cleared up whatever paperwork I had sitting on my desk. Then, I sat at my desk for a few minutes, thinking. Do I really want to go into my boss's office? Do I want to run the risk of losing possibly the best job I ever had? The answer was, that I had no other choice. My boss had a right to know what was happening to me. I was his Asst. Director, and he depended on me. So, I slowly made my way to the boss's office to speak with him, and to explain what was happening with me. I explained to my boss that I had to admit myself into the hospital, because the doctor believed that I might have cancer. I was very nervous about this, because this was a new job, and I was still on probation. I hoped this would not cause me to lose my job, but I had to be honest, even if it meant losing a job that I really enjoyed! My boss said that it would be ok, as long as I kept him informed as to my condition, and as to when I would be returning to work. Breathing a sigh of relief, I locked my office, and drove home to speak to my wife and son. On the way home, I started crying again. I loved my family, and the thought of leaving them was too much to bear. How could I possibly explain it to them? I really don't understand it, much less believe it, myself.

When I arrived home, it was very difficult explaining to my wife and seven-year old son what was happening. I told my wife first. With tears in my eyes, I told her that she had to drive me to the hospital. She said, "Why Tony? What's wrong?" I sat down, and related to her everything that the Oncologist had told me, including the biopsy that they had to perform. She asked, "How long will you be in the hospital?" I replied, "I don't know. I don't know. Honey, she said that I have cancer! I don't want to die!" I broke down and started to cry again. My wife and I just sat on the bed for a while hugging each other. Then, she helped me to pack my bag for my hospital stay. We told our son that I had to go to the hospital for some tests, and I would be there for a few days. We thought it best to wait until the tests were completed to find out exactly what was wrong with me, and what it would mean for us as a family, before we told him exactly what was going on. We called my wife's mother, explained what was happening, and she agreed to watch our son for us. So, we dropped him off at my mother-in-law's home. Then, with uncertainty and a lot of questions, my wife and I drove to the hospital. We parked the car, and went into the hospital to register. We had to wait for a while in the registration area until my room was ready. Then, someone came for me with a wheelchair. I got in, and they wheeled me to the elevator, and right up to my room, with my wife following close behind.

My wife had the forethought to call an elder from our Kingdom Hall, and explain to him that I was being admitted to the hospital, and I had not yet filled out my Health Care Power of Attorney. This is a form now requested at every hospital. It allows the patient to put in writing specific health care instructions. In my case, it provided specific instructions about the use of blood, blood fractions, and use of my own blood. It also explained whether I wished to prolong my life if my condition is considered hopeless, as well as my wishes regarding organ transplantation. This document legally takes effect only after I become unable to make or to communicate my health-care decisions myself, and it also assists the doctor when planning my treatment. Also, in the event that I am unable to do so, it allows me to appoint a health-care agent, someone who will make health-care decisions for me in the event I am unable to do so. It also serves to protect any health-care provider from legal liability when acting in accordance with my directions as expressed in my Health-Care Power of Attorney. Indeed, they are legally obligated to respect my expressed wishes. This, therefore, is a very critical document to have. So, when we arrived at my room, the elder was there waiting for us. He stayed for about three hours, explaining to my wife and I the entire document, so that I could make informed, intelligent decisions on my health-care wishes. After completing the form, it requires two witnesses to sign the document. Their signatures confirm that they witnessed me actually signing the document. So, the elder would be one witness. A nurse came over to the room and introduced herself. The elder explained the document to her, and asked if she would be the second witness, and she agreed. Then, she made several copies, one for the hospital, one for my wife and I, and one for the elder to keep in our records. She then said that she was on the floor for the remainder of the evening, and I should feel free to call her if I needed anything. We thanked her for her time and assistance. She explained that I was not scheduled for testing or anything this evening, so I could change into my pajamas, hop into bed and relax. She also said that she would call down to the kitchen and have them bring me up something to eat. The elder said that it was time for him to go, so we thanked him for his assistance. Together the three of us prayed to Jehovah God, thanking Him for watching over us, and for providing "power beyond what is normal" to help us to get through whatever adversities we may face in the near future due to my fight with cancer. After he left, I undressed, put on a pair of pajamas, and hopped into bed. My wife and I read through the information provided in the room, such as how to use the phone, and the television, and what the charges would be. A nurse came in and checked my vital signs. She then rattled off a list of medication that my doctor had prescribed for me. She handed me little white cups with pills in them, and a glass of water. She also gave me a printout for each medication, and my wife noted in her book everything the nurse said. The nurse then informed us that my doctor would be in sometime in the morning to explain the biopsy procedure. My wife and I talked until visiting hours were over. Then, she tenderly kissed me, and left to pick up our son from her mother's house. The two of them went home.

My wife returned the next morning, but I didn't see her. I didn't even realize that she was there. I had lost consciousness, and had a high fever. My wife thought, "This is it, my husband is dying!" She went into the bathroom and cried for a while. Then, she helped the nurses to put cold, wet cloths on my forehead. A friend had also stopped by to see me, but I didn't even know he was there. He stayed for a little while, and then he left. My wife stayed with me all day, until visiting hours were over. Then she left to go home. I didn't even know that she was there. I didn't know what happened the whole day, other than what my wife was able to tell me the next day. The fever finally broke, and whatever treatments I received must have worked.

I awoke the next morning to see my doctor smiling down at me. "How are you today, Tony?" she asked. "OK, I guess." I replied. My fever was gone, and I felt better. The doctor then informed me that I was well enough for her to perform the biopsy. She said that the biopsy was necessary in order to confirm what was wrong with me. She said that she would begin the biopsy in about an hour. So, I washed up, ate breakfast, and waited. The doctor and a nurse returned about an hour later to begin the biopsy. "Are you ready Tony?" the doctor asked. "As ready as I will ever be." I replied. The doctor said that she was very good at this procedure, and assured me that it would not hurt. Then, she explained again exactly what they were going to do. I was then asked to pull my pants down below the hip, and to lie on my side. As I was doing that, I noticed them preparing two large needles. One was full of something like Novocain. I received a couple of shots to numb the hip area so that I would not feel any pain. I felt a little pain with each shot, but I am a man, and it's common knowledge that men don't feel pain, so I did not say anything. Then, she used the other needle to go into my hip and withdraw some bone matter. The nurse then took this needle and prepared slides of the extracted bone matter. When they felt they had a sufficient sample of bone matter, they were finished. The doctor was pretty good, for, just like she promised, I experienced very little pain. So, they bandaged the site, and said that I could get dressed. So, I pulled up my pajama bottoms, and sat up in bed. I was told not to get the bandage wet for several days.

Then, I decided to speak to the doctor about yesterday, for I was still somewhat confused. "How come I don't remember anything that happened yesterday?" I asked. The doctor then explained to me what had happened. I don't remember everything that she said. What I do remember is that my red blood count had dropped from the normal 13–17 range, down to about 6.5. My kidneys were failing because they could not handle the large amount of proteins and excess calcium being produced by the cancer. These, and other complications, had caused the high fever, and made me lose consciousness. I was not willing to try to sustain my life by taking a blood transfusion, and my religious stand was nonnegotiable. My wife and I are Witnesses of Jehovah

God. We highly respect and value life as a gift from the Creator, and are determined not to violate His standards. We attempt to find the best in medical care and nutrition, and are willing to take medical alternatives that our conscience will allow. As a result, instead of blood transfusions, Erythropoietin and iron dextran were used to raise my red cell count, and saline solutions were used to increase blood volume. Erythropoietin is a hormone produced by the kidneys, which stimulates bone marrow to form red blood cells. I received by injection a synthetic form of this. The iron dextran was given intravenously. I received a lot of fluids intravenously to help flush the kidneys, and remove some of the toxins from my system. After explaining all of this, the doctor said that they might have the results of the biopsy later that day. She and the nurse then left the room.

My wife came in about an hour later, and she was extremely happy to see that I was up and moving around. I had given her quite a scare yesterday. We hugged each other, and I shared with her all of the information I received from the doctor. Then we discussed what we needed to do while I was in the hospital, because neither one of us knew how long I would be in there. My wife had also brought along my son Nicky, and it was really great to see him. Since she had him with her, she could not stay as long. The three of us talked for a while. Then, we went for a walk, touring the seventh floor of the hospital. I was still on intravenous fluids, so I had to push my IV pole along, but I didn't care. It was great to be together as a family again, even if only for a short time. Then, my wife and son had to leave. After they left, I laid in bed, wondering what the future held for me, and for my family.

I tried to get used to sleeping in a hospital. It was my first time sleeping in an adjustable bed, and it was difficult to find just the right setting to accommodate a sore hip, a chest with a long catheter line hanging down, and an arm full of needles. Someone from the nursing staff would come into the room every three hours to check my vital signs. It's like having a newborn baby at home. You don't actually go to sleep, you just take short naps. I was also being treated and assisted by my Primary Care Physician, my Oncologist, and a Cardiologist, so I never knew when to expect a visit. I also had to get used to hospital food. I am not saying that hospital food is bad. It's just different. I have always been a very active person—always busy, always involved in something. I just could not get used to sitting in a hospital bed doing nothing. I flipped through the channels on the television, and then turned on the music for a while while I did some reading. I had brought with me a Bible and some study materials. Finally, I drifted off to sleep.

The next morning, someone came into my room pushing a wheelchair. I asked, "Are you here to take me out for breakfast, or maybe a stroll around the park?" "No," he replied, "Your doctor has requested some x-rays, so I am taking you down to the X-ray Dept." I hopped into the wheelchair, and he wheeled me down for x-rays. He left me in the hall with my chart until the technician could see me. In about five minutes, the x-ray technician called me in, and asked me to strip to my underwear, and put on this gorgeous hospital gown with no back. When I was ready, she said that she needed to take x-rays of me from head to foot. All together, I think it was about 36 x-rays, so I was there for a while. When she was finished, she called "Transportation". It was their responsibility to wheel me around the hospital. She then wheeled me back out into the hall to wait for "Transportation" to take me back up into my room. When we got there, my wife was waiting for me. "Where have you been?" she asked. "I was out touring the hospital." I replied. Then I explained to her that they had just x-rayed me from head to foot, and that my doctor should have the results this afternoon. My wife had stopped and purchased a salad for herself, and she was hungry, so she began eating that. My lunch arrived shortly after, so my wife and I talked as we ate. I really enjoyed her company, and I missed my son.

My doctor arrived later that afternoon with her nurse practioner, and they sat down with my wife and I to talk. The doctor explained that the bone biopsy confirmed what she had already guessed, that I had Multiple Myeloma, an incurable form of bone cancer. It causes an abundance of plasma cells and immunoglobulins in the blood, contributing to kidney failure and anemia, to name a few things. It also causes bone degeneration. The X-rays showed that the cancer had already affected my bones. They found lesions, or holes, in some of the bones. My spine was degenerating, so I had several compression fractures in my lower back, and I had lost an inch in height. "So, what's the next step?" we asked. The doctor said that she was referring me to a surgeon to have a catheter installed in my chest, so that she could begin chemotherapy. She then asked if we had any questions. I had heard about catheters and probes, so I asked her which was best. She replied that a probe had more risk of infection, and she recommended a catheter. We did not have any more questions, so we thanked the doctor, and the doctor and the nurse practitioner left the room. The Oncologist was just incredible. When she asked if we had any questions, she didn't do it as she was walking out the door. She stood there and waited for a reply. If it took a few minutes for us to phrase the question, she would patiently wait. She seemed to really care about me as a person, rather than a patient, and the nurse practitioner was the same way. They were both extremely knowledgeable about the cancer field, and were able to answer intelligently, and in plain English, all of our questions. Having the two of them in my corner made a very unpleasant situation much more bearable. I cannot thank them enough for their efforts and concern in our behalf. There were a lot of things running through our minds, and we couldn't put them into words to ask the doctor. My wife kissed me and left to get our son. I sat in the room for the rest of the day, thinking. I felt that there were a lot of things I had to do, to prepare my family and myself in case the worst, my death, would actually occur. I was originally admitted to the hospital on May 6, and was released on May 18, 1999 when I was well enough to go home and prepare for the catheter installation on May 23. My wife and son came to pick me up, and I gave them both a hug. It was great to be in street clothes again, with the prospect of eating real food again with my family! We drove home, talking and laughing, happy to be together again. I had an appointment for Tuesday May 23 for the surgeon to install the catheter.

When we arrived home, my wife and I discussed what impact my having cancer, and being in the hospital, would have on our family. We also went on the Internet, and looked up "Multiple Myeloma". Multiple Myeloma is a cancer of the bone marrow that unfortunately remains incurable today. About 15,000 new individuals in the United States are affected each year, and about 50,000 total patients have Myeloma at any one given time. The 5-year survival rate has been 10–25%. The average survival time has been 24 to 30 months. Eighty percent of M.M. cases usually occurred after age 60. Although African-Americans have a significantly higher incidence rate of Myeloma as compared to those of European or Asian descent, in my age group (45–49) the risk of contracting Myeloma was about 3 cases per 100,000 persons. What really upset us was when we read that there is no cure for Multiple Myeloma. The article stated that medications could help with the pain and make you feel better, but as yet, there was no medication, no drug, that could put the cancer cells on the run, driving them out of the body once and for all. The article also stated how important it was to try and stay active, to help keep the calcium in your bones instead of in your blood. Yet, these seven words kept returning to haunt me—THERE IS NO CURE FOR MULTIPLE MYELOMA! That meant that I was dying! There was absolutely nothing the hospital could do to prevent that. It was a very difficult pill for me to swallow. I had the impossible task of preparing my family for the time when I would no longer be with them. This was extremely hard for me, because I was not prepared for it myself! I was not prepared to die, and I was not prepared to leave my family!

So, first I discussed with my wife what we needed to do in case I die. There were things I wanted to teach her. We just needed more time! I didn't want to die and leave her alone. We reviewed the will to make sure that it was current. We had our wills done by a very professional law firm. They made a separate will for me, one for my wife, gave us originals, and kept copies of the documents in their office.

Then, we talked to our children, one at a time, beginning with Nicholas, who at the time was six years old. We sat down, and I slowly began sharing with him what was wrong with me. He had heard of cancer before from television, so I tried to explain to him what it meant in my case. When we began telling him that I might die, and what that would mean for the family, Nicholas began to cry, "I don't want you to die, daddy!" he cried. I motioned for him to come to me, because my back was too weak now to pick him up, and I gave him a nice, long hug, for I was crying too. "I don't want to die either, son," I replied, "but there is a chance that I might. I need you to be prepared for it in case that I do. After all, you will become the man of the house, and I need for you to be strong, for mom and for yourself. Do you think that you can do that?" He replied, "I will try very hard to, Dad." I gave Nicholas another long hug, and then my wife and I finished our discussion with him. Nicholas was the only one of our four children still living with us, so we called the others, one by one, so that I could speak to them individually.

Our daughter, Stacey, was the oldest child, she was 25, and so we wanted to speak to her first. I began, "Stacey, I realize that I wasn't around much for you while you were growing up. I know that you perceived me as being very hard on you. I just wanted the very best for you, and I tried very hard to protect you from bad experiences, experiences that I had seen happen to people I went to school with, and people I worked with. I was always working, trying hard to support my family, and to make ends meet. I am very sorry about that, for I spent very little time at home with my children. I love you very much. I have always loved you. You are our only daughter." We hugged each other for a few minutes, and then we continued our discussion with tears in our eyes. "Now, the doctor tells us that I have cancer, and there is no cure for it. I don't know how much longer I will be around, and I will probably be spending a great deal of time in the hospital. We need you to be prepared for what might happen. Please do what you can to help mom while I am gone." Stacey replied that she would, and, through the tears, we finished our discussion with her.

Then, we prepared for our discussion with Peter, our oldest son, who was 23 years of age. The reality of losing his father was a real shock to him, but he took it well, and said that he would be there to help whenever needed, and that he would be there to take care of mom when I was gone. He then had a discussion with his wife, Monique, about the possible death of his father, and the immediate effects that the cancer would have on the family. There were personal issues involved in the relationship between my son Stephen, who was 18, and I (enough for a book all its own), so mom took care of the discussion with him. Then, for the remainder of the weekend, Shirley and Nicholas spent time with me—playing video games, board games, and having family bible studies.

On Tuesday, after driving my son Nicholas over to her mother's house, Shirley and I drove to the hospital to have the catheter installed in my chest. We parked the car, walked into the hospital, signed in, and patiently waited until my name was called. A nurse invited me back to the changing area, and asked me to take all of my clothes off, including my underwear, and to put on one of those fancy hospital gowns with the "air conditioned" back. When I was ready, she escorted me to a bed to await the surgeon and anesthesiologist. The surgeon arrived momentarily, and explained the procedure I was about to undergo to me. He asked if I had any questions. The only question I had was "Why me?" but I knew that he didn't have an answer to that, so I told him that I didn't have any questions. He said to just lay back and relax, and the anesthesiologist put me to sleep. Then, the surgeon cut a small hole in my neck, and in the left side of my chest. One end of the catheter tube was threaded into a large artery, and the other end was left hanging out of the hole in my chest. Then, the incisions were stitched up, and a large patch was placed on the incision in my chest. When I awoke, the surgeon said that the procedure went well, and asked how I was feeling. I replied that I was feeling OK, but my chest was a little sore. He explained that, in order to feed the tubes through the incisions, it causes some bruising. They had to do it twice because they were not successful in threading the catheter through to the artery the first time. He also said that dried blood had accumulated in the area, and would probably drain from the site for the next several days. The doctor then left, and a nurse informed me that I should lay there until the anesthesia wore off, and then I could get dressed. When I felt well enough to dress, my wife had to assist me. She helped me to the car, and we drove home.

At home, I showed my wife and son the catheter line hanging from my chest. It was very strange having that plastic line hanging from my chest, but it was supposed to be for my benefit, so I was willing to put up with it. I was tired, so I went to bed early. When I awoke the next morning, my pajama top was soaked with blood. Alarmed, my wife called the surgeon's office. She was informed that dried blood would drain from the area for the next several days, and she should not be alarmed. My top was soaked with blood for the next four days, so I mentioned it to the nurse practitioner at my Oncologist's office. She recommended that I make an appointment with the surgeon to have it checked. So, I made an appointment to see the surgeon. He examined it, said everything was fine, and had a fresh bandage put on. He also had a nurse show my wife and I how to flush the catheter daily to keep the line open and clear. We waited another week, and then I was read-mitted into the hospital to begin chemotherapy treatments. I was given what was termed "low-dose combination" chemotherapy. It was termed "combination" because several drugs were used in combination to fight the cancer. I believe they were termed VAD—vincristine, dex-amethesone, and doxorubicin. I remember the first time I was released from the hospital after chemotherapy treatment. I asked my wife to drive straight to my favorite pizza place to get my favorite pizza—pep-peroni and hot peppers. She did, and I couldn't wait to get it home. I ripped open the box, grabbed a piece, burning my hand and my mouth, but I didn't care. I desperately wanted some real food. To my surprise, I couldn't taste the pepperoni, the hot peppers, or even the pizza, because chemotherapy had affected my taste buds. I was eating one of my favorite foods, and I could just as well have been eating a piece of cardboard! I also began experiencing other side effects of the chemotherapy treatment, except I didn't lose my hair.

Then, I went back to the hospital for more chemotherapy treatments. My hospital stay this time was from June through October 1999. My wife was there every day, talking with me, taking notes on what the doctors and nurses said, and recording the test results. The doctors and nurses at the hospital were just great, as well as the rest of the staff. They seemed to go out of their way to assist my wife and I. My younger brother Andy flew in from Phoenix, Arizona for a surprise and very welcome visit! I just stepped out of my bathroom one afternoon, and there he was, standing in my hospital room, smiling! It was great to see him again! He and I had shared a bedroom together growing up, and we were very close. His being there, and the daily visits of my wife and son, helped me to stay positive.

Though the low-dose chemotherapy was somewhat effective in putting a hold on the progression of my cancer, my condition was not improving. I was informed by my Oncologist that it might be possible for me to live longer if I were willing to undergo a bone marrow transplant or stem cell transplant. I was also advised that this would involve blood transfusions. As was already mentioned, I am one of Jehovah's Witnesses, and my conscience would not permit me to accept blood transfusions, or any procedure involving the use of blood. My Oncologist then informed me that a bone marrow transplant was not recommended in my case. She did recommend a peripheral stem cell transplant, but she was not willing to perform the procedure without the use of blood. She said that she was very sorry, but she could not just sit there and watch me die. My wife and I were not sure what to do now. The doctor we were relying on to keep me alive could not do the procedure that would help to keep me alive because of *her* convictions, and I could not permit her to do the procedure her way because of my convictions.

So, we called and spoke to the Presiding Overseer of our congregation, and the elders from the Hospital Liaison Committee who had been assisting us up to this time. They referred us to Dr. Patricia Ford in Philadelphia. She was the only doctor on the whole East Coast, that I was aware of, to have successfully performed the peripheral stem cell transplant that I needed, without the use of blood. So, my wife and I got in touch with Dr. Ford's office, as well as the Center for Bloodless Medicine and Surgery at the Pennsylvania Hospital in Philadelphia. After checking, the office called us, and confirmed that I was accepted as a candidate for the procedure. The next step was to ensure that my health plan would cover the procedure. An RN from Dr. Ford's office did most of the legwork in preparing the necessary forms, and calling between her office and my insurance company, trying to ensure coverage for the procedure. She was very polite and efficient, doing everything she could to explain why I had to have the procedure, and why I had to go to Philadelphia. The decision of the insurance company was that Dr. Ford was not on the list of participating providers (I had an HMO), so I needed to find a doctor within the network to perform the stem cell transplant. If I insisted on using Dr. Ford, they would only pay 10% of the charges, and I would be responsible for the rest. So, the RN had desperately tried to reason with the insurance company, but to no avail. So, now it was my turn. With numerous calls and letters to the insurance company, I explained that there was not a single doctor within the network that had performed the operation successfully without the use of blood. One doctor had stated that, although he had never done it, he was willing to give it a try. I was not interested in being a guinea pig, especially since Dr. Ford had already performed the operation successfully on a number of patients without the use of blood. I advised them that I totally understood their requirements for using doctors within the network, and I had always followed this requirement without exception. This was one time, however, that I could not. I explained that, because of my religious convictions, I could not accept or use blood under any circumstances, even if my death were the only other option. I also explained that they were slowly killing me by prolonging a necessary procedure. The insurance company finally agreed to make a one-time exception, and cover the procedure. I was extremely grateful for their decision.

To explain the procedure, stem cells, also called the "mother cells", reside in the bone marrow. They divide and grow to produce three main types of blood cells—red blood cells, white blood cells, and platelets. Although the greatest concentration of stem cells is in the bone marrow, some stem cells can also be found in the circulating, or peripheral, blood stream. It is from here that the stem cells are removed, frozen, and saved for later use. High-dose chemotherapy is then administered to destroy as much of the cancer cells as possible. Unfortunately, this high-dose chemotherapy can also destroy bone marrow. Then, the stem cells are thawed and restored to the bloodstream intravenously, where they can produce whatever components of blood the body needs, and the bone marrow is regenerated. So, I was in and out of the hospital in Pittsburgh for the month of November, my Oncologist desperately trying to reduce the amount of cancer cells in my system. Then, on December 5, 1999 my wife and I were flown, free of charge, to Philadelphia, PA by a pilot who volunteers his time and his plane for cancer patients who need transportation to hospitals in other cities. This is a fantastic service, provided free of charge by people who don't want recognition or money. Their desire is simply to help, whomever they can, and they are very happy when they can provide assistance during the difficult times in a fellow human being's life. It was the first time my wife had ever flown in an airplane. A close friend drove us to meet the pilot at Allegheny Airport, and we walked over to his plane. When we initially called them, they asked us how much my wife and I weighed, insisting that we be honest and as accurate as possible with our weights. They also informed us that we could only take one suitcase each. The pilot needed to make sure that the weight limit for his plane, a four-seater, was not exceeded. I sat in the front seat with the pilot. My wife sat in one of the rear seats, and our luggage occupied the other seat. The pilot gave each of us headsets, so we could talk to each other. The flight lasted for several hours, and it was very interesting observing the different controls, gauges and instruments that the pilot used to fly the plane. The scenery was breathtaking. The pilot talked to us from time to time, explaining where we were, and what we were looking at. When he checked in and received direction from flight towers that he passed, we could hear the conversation, though we didn't understand all of it. When we arrived at the airport in Philadelphia, we thanked the pilot for selflessly giving up his time and resources to assist us in getting to Philadelphia. He replied that he was glad he was able to help, and prepared his plane for the trip back to Pittsburgh.

Someone from the Center for Bloodless Medicine and Surgery then met my wife and I at the airport. He introduced himself, took our luggage, and drove us to our hotel. It was a beautiful four-star hotel, and our room was actually a suite, with bedroom, living room, and kitchen. Our hotel room had been arranged for us by the Center, but it was being paid for by a Cancer Agency that arranges with hotels for free accommodations for cancer patients that need to travel for treatment. Our escort helped us to check in, and then carried our luggage up to the room, for I was not able to lift anything over 5 lbs. He then took us out to a shopping center to get a bite to eat. Then, we returned to the hotel to get some sleep. The next morning, our escort from the Center picked us up, and drove us to the Pennsylvania Hospital. We spoke with the people at the Center for a while, and they explained the part that they were to play in the procedure that I was about to undergo. Then, someone escorted my wife and I over to the hospital admitting area, so I could be admitted into the hospital and assigned to a room.

From December 6 through December 9, 1999 my wife and I were in the Pennsylvania Hospital in Philadelphia, where they surgically installed a catheter in the left side of my chest so that I could undergo the peripheral stem cell harvest. They removed the stem cells from my bloodstream and froze them. Then, when I was strong enough to travel, we returned to Pittsburgh to wait until my blood count returned to a satisfactory level in order to complete the stem cell transplant. My brother Ricky flew in from Papua, New Guinea, to assist me in getting some of the things that I would need for my stay in Philadelphia. We drove around to several shopping malls, looking for winter clothing. The stem cell transplant was to happen in the dead of winter, and this year, winter was worse in Philadelphia that in Pittsburgh. First, we went looking for a winter coat. We found a beautiful, red and black, very long down-filled coat. It had a big, comfortable hood that covered the head and the face. Rick paid for it, and we went next to look for a comfortable pair of boots. We found them, in addition to some comfortable white socks. My brother also bought me a thick pair of leggings. By this time, I was exhausted, so my brother drove me home, and he went on the hunt for underwear and pajamas for me. When he returned, we both had a good laugh. He had purchased a package of bikini briefs for me, the kind that is nothing more than a string in the back, and very little in the front. He had also purchased a pair of Scooby Doo boxer shorts, and a shiny pair of silver boxer shorts. He had also purchased some "real" underwear, so I was OK. This was also the perfect opportunity for him to purchase some of his favorite Pittsburgh foods, foods that were unavailable to him in Papua, New Guinea. So, we went to the different restaurants, purchased his favorite foods, and sat at home, eating, drinking, and talking. It was great to be able to spend time with him. It was difficult to do this as often as we would have liked, due to the enormous distance between our locations. He said that he would stay in Pittsburgh with us until it was time to go to Philadelphia. He would then drive to Philadelphia, and meet my sister Jackie, who was flying in from Aiken, S.C. Both of them would stay with us as long as they could while we were in Philadelphia. This was very good news.

In Pittsburgh, my kidneys failed as the Multiple Myeloma started to aggressively take over again. I was rushed to Shadyside Hospital for chemotherapy treatments. I also had to undergo albumin pheresis for the kidneys. This is something like dialysis, where my blood flowed from the catheter in the left side of my chest through a machine that removed the protein buildup that was causing my kidneys to fail. Then, the cleaned blood flowed from the machine into the catheter in the right side of my chest. This allowed my kidneys to work properly once again. This machine became an extension of my circulatory system, and I went through this procedure four times. On one occasion, my brother Rick went out to his favorite seafood restaurant and purchased fish sandwiches and fries for my wife, the nurse, himself, and me. We all had fun eating and talking while the pheresis machine did its job. After the pheresis procedures had been completed, I was informed by the nurse practitioner that a Foley catheter had to be installed to assist with my kidney function. I said, "Wait a minute! I already have two catheters, one in each side of my chest. Where is this new one going to go, in my back?" The nurse practitioner responded, "Tony, you really don't want to know." Just then, a nurse came into my room pushing a tray full of stuff and asked, "Well, Tony, are you ready?" "Ready for what?" I asked. "I am sure your doctor advised you. I need to insert this catheter into your penis." Yikes! I really DIDN'T want to know where that third catheter was going! He explained that a Foley catheter is a thin, flexible, hollow tube that is inserted through the urethra (passageway in the penis though which urine leaves the body) into the bladder. A balloon on the end is inflated with sterile water, preventing the catheter from slipping out. Urine is collected in a bag on the other end of the tube. So, I had to remove my pajama bottoms and underwear. Then, when I was ready, the nurse said for me to inhale. As I did, he held my penis, and pushed the catheter through to my bladder. The balloon was inflated to keep it in place, and a urine bag was placed on the side of my bed. Now, they were able to give me a lot of fluids intravenously, and the catheter allowed for the fluid's release. Of course, they had to empty the fluid bag a lot!

Yet, despite this and the other efforts of my Oncologist, my condition continued to worsen. So, she called the Oncologist in Philadelphia, explaining that it was critical for me to return to Philadelphia to complete the procedure. In Philadelphia, they were concerned that I was not ready to begin the procedure. My Oncologist said, "I will GET him ready. It is becoming increasingly difficult to keep the cancer in check. Please, for the welfare of my patient, schedule the procedure." I thought to myself, "I wonder how much longer I will be alive?" I did not, however, discuss this with my wife. So, my Oncologist "got me ready", and stage 2 of my transplant procedure was scheduled. I remained in the hospital, undergoing chemotherapy treatments and pheresis. I was also given iron dextran to boost my red count. I was always given a slow "push" of benadryl prior to the iron dextran, and I remember on one occasion that this did not happen. My brother Rick had come to Pittsburgh to help bolster my spirits, and to help purchase some clothing I would need for the hospital, and for Philadelphia. He was in the hospital room with me, when a relatively new nurse came in to give me the benadryl prior to the iron dextran. A doctor had to be in the room for a test dosage of the iron dextran. It is given intravenously, and he sits and watches in case the patient has a reaction to the medication. This had already been done, and the IV was already set up. The doctor had left, and the new nurse came in to "push" the benadryl through the IV tube, before the iron dextran was to begin. Unaware that this was to be slow, she pushed the entire amount through all at once, and then she left the room. When all of the benadryl hit my system at once, I found myself unable to breath, or to talk. Scared to death, I frantically motioned to my brother that I couldn't breathe, and he pushed the call button for the nurse. Then, he went out into the hall to flag down a doctor or nurse. A nurse came in quickly. I don't remember what she did, but I was extremely grateful when I was able to breathe again. I was also grateful that my brother had been in the room with me. Had he not been there, I don't know if I would have gotten assistance in time. I thought that I could have died. From that point on, I always watched everything going on. I asked questions, and made sure I understood every procedure. Mistakes can happen, and doctors and hospital staff do everything they possibly can to ensure that they don't. On the slim chance that an accident may happen, the more you know, and the more you get involved in your treatment, the less chance of a mistake happening to you.

My wife and I returned to Philadelphia on January 17, 2000. We were sitting in the hospital admittance waiting area, waiting to be called, when I stood up to go to the bathroom. I became very dizzy and lightheaded, and quickly sat back down. I said to my wife, "I guess I won't be going to the bathroom." Then, I passed out. When I woke up, I was in a gurney with tubes in my arm. My wife said that, when I passed out, they immediately sent nurses down with a gurney to help me. They determined why I passed out, started intravenous fluids, and wheeled me up to the floor I would be "living" on. My room wasn't ready yet, so I was sitting just outside the room in the hall. When the room was ready, my wife and I moved in. My brother Rick had paid for a hotel room for us, but I became too ill to leave the hospital. They provided a portable bed for my wife, and she stayed with me in the hospital room. This was necessary, because it got to the point where I could no longer take care of myself.

First, they started high dose chemotherapy, to destroy my bone marrow, and as many cancer cells as possible. I had gone through months of chemotherapy in Pittsburgh, and I had experienced various side effects. I experienced diarrhea, upset stomach, inability to taste food, etc. One thing I did not experience was hair loss, so I didn't have to experiment with hairpieces and hats. During this process of high-dose chemotherapy in Philadelphia, my red blood count dropped to 5 (normal is 13 to 17). I experienced breathing problems, and I passed out at least six times. I would be sitting in bed talking to my wife, when suddenly, I would have difficulty catching my breath. The next thing I knew, I would be waking up, and my wife would tell me how I had hit my head on the hospital post, or I had almost fallen out of the bed. I also experienced diarrhea, loss of appetite, and heart problems. I was placed on a heart monitor, and had to get breathing treatments. They could not seem to pinpoint why I was passing out. I became so weak that my wife had to help me to get out of bed, brush my teeth, shave and bathe. I was experiencing so many complications, and had become so weak, that they needed to monitor my condition around the clock. I was moved to the intensive care unit for about four days. There they connected me to so many tubes and wires and machines that I had to call a nurse for assistance just to go to the bathroom. It was difficult to find a comfortable position to lie in, but I was in so much pain and discomfort that it really didn't seem to make any difference. I had company every day—my wife, my brother Ricky, and my sister Jackie. It was a great pleasure not to be alone as I suffered through this. I was so weak and worn out, that I couldn't express how grateful I was to them for being there. I was hoping they knew. It was very depressing there, and Rick, Jackie, and my wife, helped to cheer me up, and encourage me, to get through this until I was able to return to my own hospital room.

After the first week of chemotherapy, I still had my hair, and I was relieved. I don't remember why, but my testicle sac had swollen to a huge size, and turned black. It hurt so much that I didn't want to move. One nurse brought in a heat compress wrapped in a warm towel, and she raised up my testicular sac, laying it gently on the warm towel. This felt a lot better, and I was able to get more comfortable in the bed. I think it had something to do with fluid retention, because my ankles had swollen too. They gave me water pills to help my body release the excess water, and used some other procedures that I don't remember. They worked, and my testicular sac eventually went back to its normal size and color. I was also placed on a special diet due to my low white cell count. My immune system was very weak, making me very susceptible to disease and infection. So, a huge machine was wheeled into my room to filter the air, and my door was closed. A sign was posted on my door, advising anyone coming into my room to wash their hands and wear a mask on their face. I was not permitted to eat fresh fruits or vegetables, nor was I permitted to have flowers in the room. The only water I was permitted to drink was bottled water. When they began the process of thawing my stem cells and restoring them to my system, my brother Rick was right there taking pictures with his digital camera. It seemed as if the whole room was filled with people in white uniforms, walking around and assisting with the stem cell procedure.

Then, one morning when I awoke, I saw hair on my pillow. Horrified, I went into the bathroom, brushed my hand through my hair, and patches of hair just fell out! Sooner than I wanted it to happen, I was bald! Despite all of this, I did not give in to depression or despair, because there were also good things happening at the same time. My wife had remembered to pack my electric razor. Due to the blood complications caused by the cancer, I was not permitted to shave with a blade razor. Blood clotting was no longer normal in my system. Although we brought the electric razor, we forgot to pack the cord. So, the nursing staff found a disposable electric razor that I could use. My lovely wife was there by my side the whole time, ever watchful, attending to my every need, taking notes of treatments, medications, etc.

Someone from the Center for Bloodless Medicine and Surgery always assisted us with flight and hotel arrangements, food shopping, whatever we needed. They also stopped in every morning to provide spiritual encouragement and to see how we were doing. The doctors, nurses and staff of Pennsylvania Hospital treated my wife and I very well, explaining procedures in detail, checking on us and attending to our needs. They treated us like family, rather than like patients. We also received frequent visits from two local congregations of Jehovah's Witnesses, and this was very encouraging to my wife and I.

One particular friend, who also used to live in Pittsburgh, visited on a regular basis, and helped my wife with shopping, laundry, and other things. She brought get-well cards and balloons. On one occasion, she cheered us up with two dolls, one was a spring chicken, and the other was an old goat wearing glasses. You can guess which one was supposed to be me, and which was supposed to be my wife. The three of us had a good laugh when we opened our present and the gift was explained to us. We had grown quite fond of Brenda, our friend from Pittsburgh, when she lived in Pittsburgh. She had become part of the family, and we were very sorry when she decided to move to Philadelphia. We made it a point to call her when we found out that we would be spending a good deal of time in Philadelphia. Brenda's unselfish, caring attitude and loving concern truly helped us to smile, and it encouraged us for the hard times ahead.

I have five remaining brothers and sisters, and they called regularly and provided financial assistance when possible. They also visited us at the hospital and at our home when possible, and this was very encouraging and heartwarming for me. My brother Rick flew in from Papua, New Guinea and my oldest sister Jackie flew in from Aiken, S.C. to spend time with me and to provide moral and financial support. My brother Andy also kept in touch and provided assistance when needed, in addition to flying in from Phoenix, Arizona to spend time with me in Pittsburgh. We remained in Philadelphia until February 15, 2000, when I was again well enough to travel. As soon as the doctor said that I would be able to leave in a few days, my wife and I wasted no time in finding transportation back to Pittsburgh. We called the Corporate Angel Network first, but unfortunately, they were not able to arrange for a flight for me when I needed it. They can also sometimes get cancer patients a seat on commercial private planes, but none were available going to Pittsburgh when we were planning to go. I called my sister next, for she worked for the airlines. She said that she was having trouble finding a flight for us, so I called the train station, and booked two tickets on the train to Pittsburgh. My sister called back a little later and informed us that she had located a Pittsburgh flight for us, so we cancelled the train tickets. My wife called the local Kingdom Hall, and made arrangements for someone there to pick us and our luggage up at the hospital, and take us to the airport. Brenda and my wife had previously packed up and shipped as much as they could to Pittsburgh ahead of us, because I was unable to carry anything, and my wife couldn't be burdened carrying three or four suitcases. We were escorted to the airport, and they waited until we received our tickets before they left. I had difficulty at the ticket counter. The ticketing agent refused to believe that my sister had arranged to have buddy passes there for us, because it was against airline regulations for buddy passes to be used in the absence of the airline employee that had arranged for them. She did not seem to want to listen to anything I had to say, even though I was slowly getting weak, and becoming dangerously close to once again passing out. So, I got on a pay phone, and called my sister at work in Pittsburgh. She explained to the ticketing agent that I was dying of cancer, that I had to have emergency treatment in Philadelphia, and that her boss had authorized the use of buddy passes in this emergency situation. Everything explained, the ticketing agent finally released our passes. We said goodbye and thanks to the friends that had driven us to the airport, checked in our bags, and slowly walked to the gate where we would be boarding our plane. My wife and I then returned to Pittsburgh to live out what was left of my life, and to get back to our eight-year-old son.

I was very excited to see him again! We hugged, and talked about the different things he had done while we were away. Boy, it was great to be back home again! I had really missed him. We had never been apart for such a long period of time before. My son said that he did not recognize me when I first got out of the car. I had lost a good deal of weight, and I was bald. The first time I went back to the Kingdom Hall for a religious meeting, I was very self-conscious. I did not like being bald. My son and I walked up to the doors, and there were about three of four couples walking up at the same time. I attempted to act normally, as if nothing was wrong, until my son blurted out rather loudly, "My father is bald!" So now, I was bald and beet red as I went in to the

Kingdom Hall! When we went inside, some of our friends had to look twice before they recognized who I was. I looked gaunt and sickly, but I was happy to still be alive. I was happy to still be able to attend meetings, and happy, indeed, to be with my family.

6

What Does The Future Hold?

As far as contracting the disease, very little is known as to how I contracted Multiple Myeloma. What IS known is how Multiple Myeloma is affecting me. Multiple Myeloma has caused the following side effects that may affect me at any time:

- HYPOCALCAEMIA—as my bones continue to weaken, the level of calcium in the bloodstream increases. This can contribute to fluid loss, dehydration, and kidney failure. The bones become thin, and can break with normal stresses of walking or lifting. Even coughing and minor falls and injuries can break bones. I have been cautioned not to attempt to lift anything over five pounds, and to be cautious about performing any type of exercise or sport.

- DEFECTIVE PLASMA CELLS—abnormal plasma cells replicate uncontrollably and suppress the growth of normal plasma cells. They produce an excessive amount of useless proteins called monoclonal proteins. Circulation of oxygen-carrying red cells is slowed due to hyper viscosity, and the work of the heart is increased. This can lead to headaches, dizziness, weakness, sleepiness, oozing from cuts, and other symptoms. I felt that this contributed to my having high blood pressure.

- INFECTIONS—because the body no longer makes normal antibodies, there is a high risk of infection, so people with colds, flu, etc. need to be avoided, including children less than 12 years of age, who are prone to be disease carriers. This particular side effect was very interesting to me, for my son is 9 years old. So, I get colds a lot. I also wash my hands a lot, and carry waterless hand cleaner with me, to help prevent the spread of infection.

- BENCE JONES PROTEINS—large amounts of Bence Jones proteins are excreted in the urine. This excess protein can damage the kidney filtration apparatus and the channels or tubules that are important in urine formation. Left unchecked, it can contribute to kidney failure, and an unhealthy buildup of poisons in the system.

- BACK PAIN—pain radiates from the back when the backbones collapse and impinge on nerves. In some cases, the spinal cord may be injured due to Myeloma masses that extend from the bone and press on the cord. I have lost an inch in height due to spinal compression, and have several compression fractures in my lower back. Also, I am having a difficult time managing my weight. I am at least thirty pounds overweight, and this contributes to the amount and intensity of the constant back pain that I feel.

During my hospital stays, I learned words that would become very familiar to me in the long months to come—chemotherapy, ports, steroids, EPO, renal failure, catheters, etc. I also learned something new during my hospital stay, that cancer is a term that means different things to different people. I had different cancer patients as roommates, and each one had a different form of cancer. Each one was undergoing a different type of treatment. I learned that cancer affects different people in different ways, and that the treatment can be different for each person. One roommate shared with me the importance of being positive through the whole thing—never giving up, never quitting, and starting each day with a smile on your face, NO MATTER WHAT! Another patient, with some form of mouth cancer, appeared to have given up. He wouldn't use the chemicals provided to gargle and keep his mouth clean, and the room smelled terrible. I learned from him what it means, and what it looks like, to give up. Situations may appear desperate at times, even hopeless. Is it worth it, though, to give up on life, or on yourself? It does no one any good, not you, not your family. Though having cancer can change your life and that of your family, I also learned that it doesn't have to mean the end of everything. Cancer is not necessarily a death sentence, and even if it is, as in my case, you can still live each and every day to the fullest, always thinking positive! Yes, we can proactively choose how we deal with the cancer that impacts our lives. We can choose not to focus on the negative things. We can choose, instead, to focus on the good things in our lives—our families, our friends, and the fact that we are still alive, TODAY! Whatever treatments we have to undergo, whatever medications we have to take, we can go through this with a smile, taking life one day at a time.

This whole ordeal has truly been a learning process for me. When I first received the diagnosis, a period of intense inner confusion and conflict began. Who do I tell? How much do I tell them? First, since I was still at work, I told my boss. Then, I went home and told my wife, crying because I could not hold back the tears. I then told each of my four children. It was difficult telling my six-year-old son, because it was difficult to determine how much he really understood. It is difficult for the children to accept the fact that their father will not be around to help them and have fun with them as they grow older. My daughter, though 26 years old, never came to see me while I was in the hospital, not even once. She never told me why, but she did try to explain it to my wife. She loved me very much, and it hurt her to see her father dying, and in so much pain. She just couldn't bear it, and could not stand seeing me in the hospital. She was not able to deal with it emotionally. Every time I returned home, though, she was right there, checking on my condition, seeing how I was doing, and seeing if I needed anything. My other two boys and my daughter-in-law were also very supportive of my wife and I. They visited and called us on a regular basis.

My son is 9 years old now, and he still cries when he hears me or someone else discussing the possibility that I may die. Once, while I was talking to my wife, preparing her for what to do if I were to die, my son started crying and saying that he did not want me to die. I couldn't pick him up, so I walked over to him, hugged him, then held him close in my arms. I again explained to him that I did not wish to die, and that I would do everything I possibly could to live as long as possible. I might die, but I would try very hard not to.

My wife was a little confused about a certain change in my leisure time. My oldest son had given my son Nicky a Super Nintendo game player, with a Super Mario Brothers game cartridge, and he begged me to play with him. I had never played video games before, and I was not interested in starting now, but I did want to spend time with my son. The condition of my bones made it virtually impossible to play with him in any other way. So, while my son was in school, I played Super Mario Brothers, hoping to understand the game well enough to play with my son when he came home from school. My wife would come down for breakfast in the morning and find me playing Super Mario Brothers. While my son was in school, I would be playing Super Mario Brothers. I had become addicted to the game, and I really enjoyed it! So, my son and I really enjoyed spending time with each other playing Super Mario Brothers. We later purchased a Sega Dreamcast, and additional games, as well as additional cartridges for the Super Nintendo, so I became somewhat proficient in video game play, though I could never hope to be as good as my young son.

Finally, I shared my health condition with family and friends. It really helped to be able to talk to other people about my illness, and my condition. It prevented me from feeling that I was all alone, and possibly giving in to the disease. I was able to speak with others who I never knew had gone through similar experiences, or worse experiences, and they were taking things one day at a time. They were happy to be alive, and happy that they were still able to spend time with their families. They were also happy that they could still spend time serving God, for it was he that provided the greatest support and encouragement, and his phone line—prayer—was always open.

Another important thing to do is to form a partnership with your doctor. I found a doctor that I could really talk to. I trusted her, and she would always take the time to make sure that my wife and I understood every procedure. She listened, and seemed to really care about her patients. Each patient was treated as an individual, and she tried to learn as much as possible about my physical, emotional, and spiritual needs, and as much trials and tribulations that my wife and I had to undergo, her kind, considerate, and caring attitude made all the difference in the world in our being able to understand and better deal with, what was going on in my life.

I also received cards, phone calls, visits, and money from fellow workers, friends and family too numerous to mention. It brought tears of joy to my eyes, realizing that I had touched the lives of so many people, and now they were here for me in my time of need. Their support and encouragement has really helped me to get through the tough times.

I have also been able to view my darling wife through different eyes. She has been there for me, with me, every step of the way. When I was depressed and gave way to tears, she was there to hold me, to comfort me. When I had diarrhea due to chemotherapy, and was too weak to take care of myself, my wife took on the terrible task of cleaning me up and changing my underwear. She also had to bathe me every morning. The nursing staff said that it was not necessary, that they would be happy to do it. I did allow one nurse to wash me up one time. When it came time to wash up my private area, I told the nurse thank you very much, but I would wait until my wife arrived to have that washed. I realized that the nurses had seen every part of my anatomy by this point, but I still felt uncomfortable with someone seeing and washing that part of my anatomy, so I waited until my wife came to do it. She said that she didn't mind. My wife was there every day at the hospital, watching, taking notes about my condition, getting things that I needed, and making sure that I ate properly. She kept the business cards provided by the different doctors, nurses, Social Workers, etc. She also took the printed information about my medications and treatments, reviewed and then filed them for me. Now that I have been released from the hospital, she has become my nurse, attending to my every need, making sure I take my medication, and giving me shots. I love her so very, very much.

I also realize that I still have a hard road ahead of me. My Oncologist accepted a teaching position in another state, so I had to start seeing another Oncologist in the practice. There is no cure yet for the cancer that I have. I was taking thalomid and steroids to try and keep the cancer in remission and it worked for a time. Then, the cancer became aggressive once again, so Cytoxan, a chemotherapy drug, was added to my monthly regimen. My wife has had to give me Neupogen shots to raise my white blood count, and Procrit shots to raise my red blood count. Once a month a nurse comes to the house to give me a four-hour injection of Aredia, which helps to reduce bone degeneration. I went through a period of depression that I could not shake, so I am also taking an antidepressant. I am fatigued and sleepy most of the time due to the Thalomid medication, so because of this and other complications, I am no longer able to hold a job. I am no longer employed by the Housing Authority City of Pittsburgh. They did everything they could for me while I was able to work. They made reasonable accommodations whenever necessary to allow me to continue working as long as I could. When I could no longer work, they were extremely helpful in assisting me with paperwork, forms, and understanding what direction to go for continued health and life insurance coverage. I worked with a lot of good people, and I was sorry that I had to leave.

I am now on Social Security Disability. The struggle to get disability could provide enough information for a book all to itself. When I initially applied for disability, I was unable to work. My Oncologist said that my bones were so fragile that I could break a bone even walking or sneezing. My immune system was low, so I had to avoid crowds. My blood was not able to clot properly, so I had to be very careful not to get a cut or wound. I applied for, and received, a handicap placard for my vehicle, but I was denied SSI Disability! I applied for Public Assistance, and was denied twice before my wife and I were finally approved. We had to hire an attorney to fight in our behalf for SSI Disability, and then he received 25% of the money that we needed to survive. Our medical coverage while on Public Assistance was great, but as soon as we qualified for SSI Disability, this was dropped, and we had to pay almost 1/3 of our disability check for medical coverage. Eventually, I was strong enough to be able to return to work. After almost a year of absence, my position as Assistant Director was still available. I worked for about a month before I notified the Social Security office. I wanted to be sure that I could work full-time. When I contacted the Social Security office, they informed me that I still had a trial work period, and they would send me a brochure to explain. When the brochure arrived, I read through it. It said that, if I returned to work, I would have a 9-month trial period where I would continue to receive checks. If I were able to continue working, the checks would continue for 3 more months, and then stop. When I noticed that the allowed time period had elapsed, I called the office to see when the checks would stop, and they said they would have to send me a form to fill out. I filled out the form completely and returned it. Soon I received a letter from them stating that I had been overpaid about several thousand dollars. My wife and I wrote letters, visited the local office, but to no avail. They still insisted that I owed them the money. At the time of this writing, I am waiting for a hearing before an Administrative Law Judge to dispute it. Then, when I realized in December 2001 that I would have to stop working, I called the local Social Security Office and notified them that I would like to start my SSI Disability payments. My wife and I were advised to come to the office to fill out paperwork, which we did. The caseworker mentioned that he was having trouble entering our check information because of the overpayment I mentioned earlier, but that shouldn't hold up my first check. He assured me that we would receive our first check March 20, 2002. If the overpayment were still a problem, he would see that an emergency check was provided. I thought everything was OK, until March 2002 arrived, and I had not received any written notification from SSI about my payments. So, I called the local office again. Another caseworker answered. He checked my account, and said that I would not receive a check until May. He put me on hold until my caseworker could investigate. A few minutes later, my caseworker came on the line and said that the overpayment had been taken out of my checks, and I would therefore not receive a check until the third Wednesday in May. I said that I had no income and no food, what were we supposed to do? He suggested that we go to the Public Assistance office. So, my wife and I went to the Public Assistance office, filled out the necessary forms, waited our turn, and were politely informed that we did not qualify for Public Assistance because we qualified for SSI Disability. When I informed her that we would not receive disability until May, she said that we needed to go back to the local SS office and request a waiver. They should not have taken all of our money. So, my wife and I got back into our car, and drove back to the SS office. On the way, we wondered why our caseworker hadn't told us any of this. When we arrived at the SS office, we were informed that our caseworker wasn't seeing people today, but the woman at the desk gave us the forms to fill out to request partial payments. Shortly thereafter, we received a letter from SSI, stating that our request for partial payments was approved, and our first check would be received April 3, 2002. When that didn't happen, I again called the local office, and I was informed that the letter was incorrect. My checks would always be received on the third Wednesday of the month. I then asked why, if I was eligible for payments as of February 2002, why was I not receiving a check until April? He checked, and replied that they held the entire March check because of the overpayment. He said if we could come to the office and fill out some more forms, he could straighten it out. My wife and I went to the office once again, talked to a different caseworker, filled out the forms, and he gave us a check for the March payment, minus the partial payment. I sincerely hope that others don't experience the same difficulties we experienced in getting the assistance we need from the government, when necessary.

I have learned through my experience with Multiple Myeloma to look at life through different eyes. I finally realized that I don't need to be a workaholic, spending all my waking hours working, or thinking about work, at the expense of my family. Now, I take things one day at a time. I no longer worry about the small things. A friend that I had worked with and started a business with was now employed by Shadyside Hospital, and he had stopped in to pay me a visit. He gave me a book, entitled *Don't Sweat the Small Stuff.* I read it with interest, and it made a lot of sense. I take time to appreciate my family, and take time out for doing fun things. We realize that each day could very well be my last, but it could also be the beginning of a long and happy life, because cancer affects each person differently. I no longer worry about cancer statistics and percentages. Each day can and will be an adventure—an adventure filled with the love and support of friends and family. Initially, I looked at myself as a cancer "victim". Cancer reared its ugly head, and slowly changed my life. I could no longer work, so I lost my position as Assistant Director. I lost my office, my company car, my laptop, my cell phone, everything. It was a job I really enjoyed, a job I was good at. Now, because of cancer, it was gone. Cancer affected my health. I would now spend a great deal of time in and out of hospitals and doctor's offices, taking all sorts of drugs and medications. I am very easily tired and, because of low immunity, I sometimes have to avoid crowds. So, I can't enjoy parks, movies, even going shopping with my wife and son. I am tired most of the time, and because of the medications, it is often difficult for me to think clearly. The cancer weakens my bones, so I can't run, play ball, or ride bikes with my son.

I can't even pick up my son or play with him. I could continue the list, but what's the point? Being a "victim", just feeling sorry for myself, just steals precious moments of time from my family, and I don't know how much time I have left. So, I now look at myself as a cancer "survivor", and take life one day at a time. Yes, I have cancer, but I am still alive! I am still well enough to enjoy the companionship of my wife and son. I am also still around for my other children if and when they need me. I still have a sense of humor, and I still have my precious relationship with God. The Center for Bloodless Medicine and Surgery at Pennsylvania Hospital in Philadelphia recently sent me their first issue of their quarterly newsletter. I found it to be very informative, and it helped to bring back positive memories of their assistance and support while I was in Philadelphia. One of their feature articles was entitled *My Struggle with Multiple Myeloma* by Anthony Luck. I enjoyed that article also.

My Oncologist recently switched to a new Health Care Organization, so I have to look for another Oncologist, and start the process all over again. I have to search for a new Oncologist, and start all over again building up a relationship with a new doctor, and a new group of health care specialists.

Nothing ever seems to go easily. Yet, I plan on being more than a cancer survivor. I look forward to the day prophesied in the Bible at Isaiah 33:24 where "no resident will say I am sick". I look forward to the time mentioned at Revelation 21:3,4 "Look! The tent of God is with mankind, and he will reside with them, and they will be his peoples, and God himself will be with them. And he will wipe out every tear from their eyes, and death will be no more, neither will mourning nor outcry nor pain be anymore. The former things have passed away." Until that day comes, I will survive. I will enjoy life, and I will enjoy my family. "If it is to be, it is up to me" and my personal relationship with God. Faith in Him and His promises keeps me going. One of these days I hope to see my father again, and we will have a lot to talk about. I think about him a lot, and I miss him very much. He was a good man, and a great father. I hope I am a lot like him. I dedicate this book to him, to keep his memory alive a little longer—for his family, his friends, and for me. I MISS YOU DADDY—VERY MUCH!

Conclusions

❖

10 Things That Cancer Patients, Their Family And Friends Should Know!

I have learned a lot during my hospital experience, and I would like to share some of this knowledge with others. Hopefully, it will help other cancer patients and their families to get through the tough times. In particular, there are things I felt that the family and friends of cancer patients should know, as well as the cancer patients themselves. So, here goes!! These 10 items, just like the information found in the rest of this book, are from my perspective, my point of view. Check with your doctor and your family to see if they may apply in your case:

1. ***NEVER GIVE UP!***—No matter what type of cancer you have, you always have a chance. There is a chance to get better, a chance to fight, and a chance you can win! Talk to your doctor often. Discuss your options, treatments, procedures, medications, etc. Research the Internet, try to understand clearly what is happening to you, and why. The more you know about your particular form of cancer, the better your chances of understanding and following the treatments. See if there are any natural supplements you can take to help keep your body functioning properly. Of course, if you are taking any type of supplements, be sure to share this with your doctor, to avoid any interactions with the medication he/she may prescribe. Also, when you apply for benefits, whether social security, disability, public assistance, whatever, never, never take NO for an answer. Fight for whatever benefits are rightfully yours. Do not get discouraged if benefits are initially denied. Don't

accept the denial. Fight for your rights and WIN! I don't know if you ever heard the story of the miners who gave up and stopped digging just inches before the biggest gold vein in history! Don't ever give up! Keep digging! Never give up on yourself, or on life itself! Fight for each day of life, for yourself, and for your family. Enjoy each day, one day at a time. Enjoy living, and enjoy your family for as long as you possibly can!

2. ***DON'T BE AFRAID TO ASK FOR HELP!***—There may be little changes in your system or habits that your doctor may need to know, such as changes in bowel movements, eating habits, how you feel, etc. Don't hesitate to share this information with your doctor or caregiver. It may just help with your treatment. In addition, the effects of the cancer you have may limit your ability to work, to do things around the house, etc. Don't be afraid to ask family and friends for assistance when needed. In most cases, they WANT to help, they just don't know HOW! Plus, there is a whole Cancer Assistance Network out there to help cancer survivors, so don't be afraid to ask for their help. For example, there are pilots who willingly donate their time and their own planes to fly cancer patients to hospitals they need to go to, at no cost to the patient. Some hotels, through the Cancer Assistance Networks, offer rooms, if available, free of charge or at minimum cost to cancer patients getting treatment away from home. There are some organizations that offer reimbursement for some medical expenses for cancer patients. There may be an organization set up for your particular form of cancer. These are just a few examples. You can get a list of organizations from the American Cancer Society, from the Internet, or possibly from the Social Worker at your hospital. There are a lot of people and organizations that are willing and able to help out when needed. So, don't be afraid to ask for help when help is needed. ASK! You would be surprised just how many organizations and support groups are out there for cancer patients and their families.

3. *BE POSITIVE!*—I know this is easy to say, and sometimes extremely difficult to do, but it is so important to do! When you are sick, it is easy to get discouraged. It is easy to feel rejected, lonely, ready to give up, etc. It is not so easy to be positive, but it is important—to your well-being, and that of your family. Wake up each and every morning with a smile on your face, and with a positive outlook. Make an effort each and every day to make it a great day! It will keep you optimistic, and it will have a positive effect on those around you! Don't dwell on the cancer, or on being sick. It will only depress you. Focus, instead, on the good things in your life—your family, your friends, and the fact that you are still alive! A positive outlook will not only make you feel better, but it will also do wonders for your family. Being negative and depressed hurts, and does no good for anyone. Being optimistic helps to strengthen you and your family. It also makes it easier for the doctors and nursing staff of the hospital to help you, and to work with you.

4. *KNOW YOUR MEDICATIONS!*—Make a list of the medications you are currently on, including the names, dosages, and frequencies. Keep this list in your wallet or purse. You never know when you may be asked what medications you are on, so it is good to have the list handy. You may have to see doctors other than your own due to complications of the cancer, and they will need to know what medications you are on. It is also extremely important to remember to TAKE your medications. It might be helpful to use a calendar, or something similar, to keep track of when, and how much, medication to take. While you are in the hospital, if medications are brought in for you to take, if you do not know what they are, ASK! Ask for a printout that describes each medication—what it is, what it is used for, what the side effects are. You have a right to know. It's good to know what you are taking, and why you are taking it. It's also good to know what the side effects may be. Remember to share this information with your family, so that they know.

5. ***KEEP GOOD RECORDS***—Use a monthly calendar (or something similar) to keep track of doctor's appointments, chemotherapy treatments, hospital stays, medications, etc. This information will be very useful when filing for disability or insurance benefits, or when filing for reimbursements. It is also good for you to make sure that scheduled treatments are done on time, and to keep track of appointments. It will be difficult at a later date for you to remember all of your previous appointments. It is also good to save receipts for reimbursement purposes.

Now these last five are primarily for friends and family.

6. ***REMEMBER THE EFFECTS OF MEDICATION!***—Always try to keep in mind that the different medications, and sometimes even the cancer itself, may make the cancer patient irritable, depressed, or a host of other moods. The cancer patient seems to become someone entirely different than the person that you used to know. Be patient, realizing that the patient is sometimes being difficult, not because they want to be, but because of the medication, or because of the cancer itself. Help the patient to get through the difficult times. Try to remain calm and relaxed, no matter what emotion the patient is going through. Remember, the patient needs your encouragement and support, never your anger.

7. ***KNOW AND UNDERSTAND WHAT THE PATIENT NEEDS TO DO, THEN HELP HIM DO IT!***—There will be a lot of instructions and information communicated during the cancer treatment process that the patient needs to keep and remember. A good note taker will be extremely helpful during this time. Then, do what you can to assist the cancer patient to follow the instructions.

8. **DON'T ASK—DO!**—Don't ask, "So, what can I do to help?"
There are normal, everyday things that need to be done that can be
done without asking:

- The family car, such as washing, vacuuming, maintenance

- Lawn care

- Sweep the porch, and the front of the home

- Wash the windows

- Empty the trash

- Housecleaning or washing clothes

- Grocery shopping

- Cooking a meal

- Taking young children to give mom a break.

It is difficult to ask for help, even when you are too ill to do things
for yourself. So, don't wait around until the cancer patient asks for
help. They may never do so. Pitch in and do what needs done.
They will thank you for it! Even if they don't, it's the right thing to
do!

9. **HOSPITAL VISITS!**—Sometimes, when a cancer patient sits
alone in their hospital room, feelings set in, such as doubts, fears,
depression, loneliness, etc. So, in most cases, visits, cards, and calls
are welcome. It's terrible to sit alone in a hospital room. Depression and feelings of loneliness become hard to shake, and it
becomes increasingly difficult to feel good about yourself, and
about life. Calls, visits and cards help to put aside those feelings,
and to help the cancer patient to think of happier things. When
you visit, though, try to be mindful of the time. Lengthy visits may
be tiring to the patient due to medication. Also, bathroom visits
may need to be more frequent due to the medication, yet difficult

or embarrassing when visitors are present. So, keep hospital visits brief, but visit often if you can.

10. ***CONSIDER OTHER FAMILY MEMBERS!***—Just as the cancer patient has needs, so do the family members, such as the spouse, and the children. Family members are often consumed with providing for the health and well being of the cancer patient. This can be very stressful. Why not find time to talk with family members? Find out what their needs are. Invite them out for some form of recreation, or perhaps invite them over to your house. Sometimes just a few hours away from worries and anxieties is just what they need to keep them going, to keep them positive, and to get them through the difficult times.

Cancer. Just the sound of that word is enough to send chills up and down your spine. I don't want to have cancer, especially a form of cancer that's terminal. Nobody does. It has really been a learning experience for me. I have learned to slow down and appreciate every day, every minute that I am alive. I have learned the importance of spending quality time with my wife and my son. For years I had been a "workaholic". Now, I realize that tomorrow is not guaranteed to anyone, so my todays are spent with my family. I don't know how much longer I have, but there is one thing I do know. I am going to enjoy every minute that I am alive. It is very difficult to enjoy life when you sit around angry or depressed because you are sick. Yes, I am sick, and I am dying, but so what? I am alive today, and today, I am going to enjoy life, and I am going to enjoy my family! Thinking about the cancer, and how it is slowly stealing my life, robbing my family and I of happiness, will not make things better. It will only serve to depress me, and depress my family. So, I don't think about cancer. Instead, I view each new day as a gift to be enjoyed, and spend every possible minute with my wife, and my children. I spend time each day reading God's word the Bible, and I thank God each day for another day of life. Cancer may be terminal, but it doesn't have to be miserable. It will be whatever you make it. If you are a cancer patient, focus on the good things in your life. If you are friend or family, be a true friend to the cancer patient. They will desperately need it. For me, I attempt to make my cancer invisible, and I focus on the important things in life. I focus on my family, my friends, and my relationship with God. The cancer may beat me physically, but mentally, spiritually, I am determined to be the winner! So, remember the positive attitude, and remember the above-mentioned ten things! Cancer sometimes wins the battle, but don't EVER let it win the war! Be strong, and remain strong, for yourself, and for your family. Be a cancer survivor for as long as you possibly can. With a strong will, loving family and friends, a doctor that you can trust, and a loving Heavenly Father, a lot of impossible things can become possible! I hope that you are able to beat your form of cancer. If it is terminal, as it is in my case, so what! Don't ever let the cancer beat you! Take things one day at a time, and be sure to enjoy your family and friends, and continue to enjoy each and every minute of life that you have. That is exactly what I intend to do! So, whatever happens, make it a good one, and always try to think positive. It will help to make whatever form of cancer that you have a little easier to bear, not only for you, but also for your family. Believe me, it will be worth the effort!

About the Author

Anthony D. Luck, happily married husband and father of four children, comes from a close family of three brothers and four sisters. When he heard the news that his beloved father was stricken with cancer and was about to die, it seemed as if his whole world had just been turned upside down. The potential loss of a parent is truly devastating. His father died not long after that, in 1988.

Then, in 1999, Anthony got the devastating news that he had Multiple Myeloma, an incurable form of bone cancer. He was also informed that Multiple Myeloma was the same cancer that took the life of his father, just eleven years ago. At the time, he was employed as an Assistant Director for the Housing Authority City of Pittsburgh. How does he tell his employer? More importantly, how does he tell his wife, his children, and his family? Now, no longer able to work, Anthony is currently on SSI Disability. He is a former member of the Speakers' Bureau, and is currently on the National Cancer Survivors' 2002 Speakers List. He was also an active participant in a program called "Choices", visiting schools throughout the area, speaking with 9th and 10th graders about how the choices that they make today affect their future, hoping to have them think twice about dropping out of school. Anthony has assisted with fundraising efforts for United Way, Spina Bifida Association, MDA, and, with this book, the International Myeloma Foundation. Now, faced with thoughts every day of losing his life the same way that his father did, and leaving his wife and children alone, Anthony has a constant daily struggle to stay positive and cheerful. With God's help, with the love and assistance of family and friends, and with the help of knowledgeable doctors and staff, Anthony hopes to beat the odds, and outlive the life expectancy of the average Multiple Myeloma patient.

0-595-22973-5

www.ingramcontent.com/pod-product-compliance
Lightning Source LLC
Chambersburg PA
CBHW031232280526
45784CB00004B/1535